TURN ON, TUNE IN, AND HEAL

Personal Stories of Healing with Psychedelics

By Alisa Stone

Turn On, Tune In, And Heal

Copyright © 2024 by Alisa Stone

All rights reserved.

Artwork by Meg Levine

ISBN: 979-8-9923053-1-9 eBook

ISBN: 979-8-9923053-0-2

Published by Open Heart

2025

Proceeds from this book will be donated to organizations working to legalize use of psychedelics, groups working to advocate for safe and inclusive practices and harm reduction education.

For bulk sales or to be put on an email list, contact the author by email:

Alisastonehealing@yahoo.com

TABLE OF CONTENTS

"They love to tell you stay inside the lines. But something's better on the other side."
- John Mayer

This book is dedicated to everyone in search of healing. Hope is something no one should ever be without, and for many, these substances have brought that hope to life, lighting a path toward healing and transformation.

I am deeply grateful to those who courageously shared their personal stories of healing to inspire others, offering a beacon of possibility when all else seemed to fail.

Thank you to my family, who supported me on this journey, even with initial concerns and uncertainties. And to the friends to whom I finally opened up to about my healing journey. Whose compassion and open hearts were there for me, even when this path was far outside their own experience.

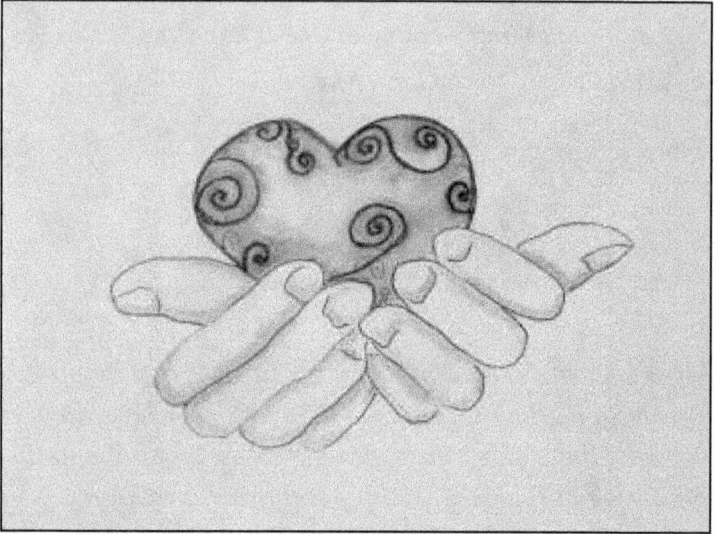

INTRODUCTION

People take different roads seeking fulfillment and happiness. Just because they aren't on your road doesn't mean they've gotten lost."
-Dalai Lama XIV "

Your banker, doctor, neighbor, and mailman are probably doing it. Maybe your accountant, or your son's school teacher. No, I'm not talking about a 5:00 PM vodka martini–I'm talking about microdosing and using psychedelics for healing. Although psychedelic use is largely kept underground due to its illegality, compelling evidence from university studies, scientific research, and clinical trials are revealing how these substances can change lives for the better.

Many cultures for thousands of years have used plant medicines like San Pedro, Peyote, Psilocybin, Ayahuasca and Cannabis for mental and physical healing, relationship improvement, and even to soothe squabbles between neighboring tribes. Plants like psilocybin, mescaline and LSD act in the brain similarly. They all have the effect of simulating 5-HT2A and increase the interaction between serotonin, BDNF, and glutamate. This can result in people developing a new perspective on things.

Drawings and artifacts of psychedelic plants found worldwide in tombs and caves show they have been used as a sacrament in healing and spiritual ceremonial traditions in the entire world except Antarctica. They have been used in the Amazon Basin, by indigenous peoples of Mexico, in Native North American communities, and in several tribes in Africa. In ancient Greece there has been evidence of psychoactive plant usage in various ceremonies. Indigenous peoples of Siberia and the Sai people of Northern Europe used mushrooms in their sacred traditions.

In the early 20th century, scientists invented MDMA and LSD in a lab with similar effects. Since their invention, there has been increased interest in the therapeutic use of psychedelics for healing, personal growth, and spiritual exploration. Many people report profound experiences and insights from their use of psychedelics, and there is a growing movement to legalize and regulate their use for these purposes in the United States. A few other countries, such as Australia, South Africa, Peru, Jamaica, and Brazil have already started using them in mainstream medicine. Some countries such as Switzerland and Israel have also legalized or decriminalized different psychedelics under the heading of compassionate use. Note this isn't a complete list, just some examples.

Psychedelics can be a beneficial therapeutic tool as they ultimately allow an individual to be detached and dispassionately look at past traumas and experiences. They allow the brain to look at and process the situations without causing the flight, fight, freeze response. This is why the claims that one psychedelic session can be equal to many years of talk therapy seem to bear out, especially when used in conjunction with talk therapy. Studies show people feel 60% "cured" just after one session, a transformation that is lingering, and sometimes permanent. After taking a few sessions with psychedelics.

Two thirds of PTSD patients no longer qualified for PTSD diagnosis. [1]

At the time of the writing of this book, most of these medicines are still identified as Schedule 1 drugs, meaning they are associated with a high risk of abuse and have no safe, accepted medical use. However, clear benefits of psychedelics have been known for centuries. In the 1950's and 60's, modern doctors and scientists were actively studying these benefits until their research was shut down and these substances were labeled as Schedule 1 substances. All studies ceased in 1968. It didn't stop the usage of psychedelics, however; it just sent it underground. But what it did was stop the official teaching hospitals and Universities from conducting trials, research, and possibly facilitating mainstream healing. Senator Robert F. Kennedy even fought to keep psychedelics legal for research in 1968, arguing, "If they were worthwhile six months ago, why aren't they worthwhile now?" Kennedy's wife, Ethel, had received psychedelic therapy

---

[1] Barbaro, Michael, et al. "The Veterans Fighting to Legalize Psychedelics." *The New York Times*, The New York Times, 22 Feb. 2023, www.nytimes.com/2023/02/22/podcasts/the-daily/veterans-psychedelics-legalization.html.

at Hollywood Hospital in Vancouver, and Kennedy argued it would be a loss to the nation if psychedelics were banned due to illicit use.

Despite being categorized as a Schedule 1 drug, public and scientific interest in psychedelic use has continued to grow over the years. Thousands of studies, trials, and research conducted at top universities worldwide have revealed how psychedelics can help people who suffer from anxiety, depression, OCD, alcoholism, prescription drug abuse, tobacco or nicotine addiction, PTSD, menstruation issues, and more. Johns Hopkins, UCLA, and NYU are even conducting studies on volunteers with end-stage cancers. Patients have reported to undergo profound spiritual experiences, under the influence of these substances, which allowed them to accept their terminal illness and confront death without fear.

Studies on psychedelics have ultimately proven them to be biologically transformative, but not physically addictive. Psilocybin mushrooms, LSD, and DMT have all been found to stimulate neuroplasticity, which allows the brain to generate new neurons and connections. MRIs have been used to track brain activity in healthy individuals under the influence of different psychedelics. These studies have revealed hyper-connectivity in the brain, which allows normally unrelated and cautious regions to communicate with each other. Psychedelics are also known to induce nerve growth factors as well. Scientists also discovered the default mode network (DMN), which is the part of the brain that you use during daydreaming or wakeful rest. It's the area used for remembering the past, envisioning the future, and self-reflection. During a 'trip' the DMN becomes disorganized which is why people feel the 'ego dissolution' - a sense that they are a part of everything. When serotonin receptors relax, one becomes happier. Comprehensive data and research on psychedelics have shown that flashbacks, long lasting psychoses, schizophrenia, or severe depression and addiction are simply scare tactics used to turn the societal tide against these substances. It is crucial to distinguish evidence-based risks from unfounded claims, inviting and allowing for informed discussions and policies surrounding their use.

In the 1980's Rick Doblin founded the Multidisciplinary Association for Psychedelic Studies (MAPS). The first scientific studies on human subjects started above ground in 2014. Since then, scientific research on psychedelics has exploded. Top universities are securing grants for their research, and some cities in the U.S. along with other countries are slowly easing their laws regarding psychedelic usage. In 2019, a study from Columbia University Irving Medical Center revealed a downward trend in negative perceptions toward LSD, in particular, estimating that over 5.5 million people had taken this substance.

LSD alone has been credited with giving individuals a boom in creativity. Steve Jobs called LSD "a profound experience, one of the most important things in my life." Kary Mullis, who invented the polymerase chain that makes cloning possible, credited his LSD use for the inspiration. Francis Crick, a molecular biologist and Nobel Prize winner, is said to have identified the double-helix structure of DNA because of an LSD trip. Ray Charles also attributed most of his hits to LSD use. Bill Wilson, the founder of Alcoholics Anonymous (AA), attributed his profound shift into sobriety to LSD. Rumor has it that Mary Shelley even penned *Frankenstein* after ingesting ergot, which is synthesized into LSD.

Over the past two years, I have collected true stories of healing from willing, generous, and brave individuals across the globe. While some stories are sourced from people in international psychedelic societies, others were contributed by individuals who heard about this project and wanted to share their own healing experiences with psychedelic use. These inspiring stories highlight the power of psychedelic therapy as a means of addressing childhood trauma, PTSD, depression, alcoholism, chronic pain, disordered eating, anxiety, OCD, and other ailments.

My intention for curating all these stories of healing is for the purpose of stigma reduction. Psychedelic therapy has taken place largely in the shadows for the past 50 years, but needs to be out in the light once again. It needs to be a mainstream conversation without the fear of ramifications from the law, or receiving judgment. This mirrors the journey of acceptance that therapies like antidepressants and talk therapy underwent in the 1970s and 1980s when many hesitated to admit to turning that direction. It's time for healing to be openly embraced.

My own story echoes countless others who have demonstrated incredible bravery in sharing their journeys with psychedelics. I am a 63-year-old woman who embraces the roles of wife, mother, friend, volunteer, and nature lover. Although I am not a scientist or doctor, my deepest aspiration is to inspire and positively impact the lives around me. Throughout my lifetime, I have explored every imaginable avenue in an attempt to heal my own wounds stemming from childhood neglect and depression. Eventually, I found solace and relief through the use of these healing substances.

The authors of these stories have heeded the words of the renowned Timothy Leary–"Turn on, tune in, and drop out"–by embracing some form of psychedelic therapy. However, they did not detach from society. Instead, they dropped back in, reconnecting with their bodies, their work, their relationships, and their communities. Together, we form a vast tapestry of individuals, spanning different ages, genders, ethnicities, nationalities, and professions. You might not suspect these authors of engaging in such practices if you knew them from work settings, professional services, or your place of worship. Yet, what unites all of us is our deep-seated desire to heal ourselves and support others on their healing journeys. I hope these stories will inspire you.

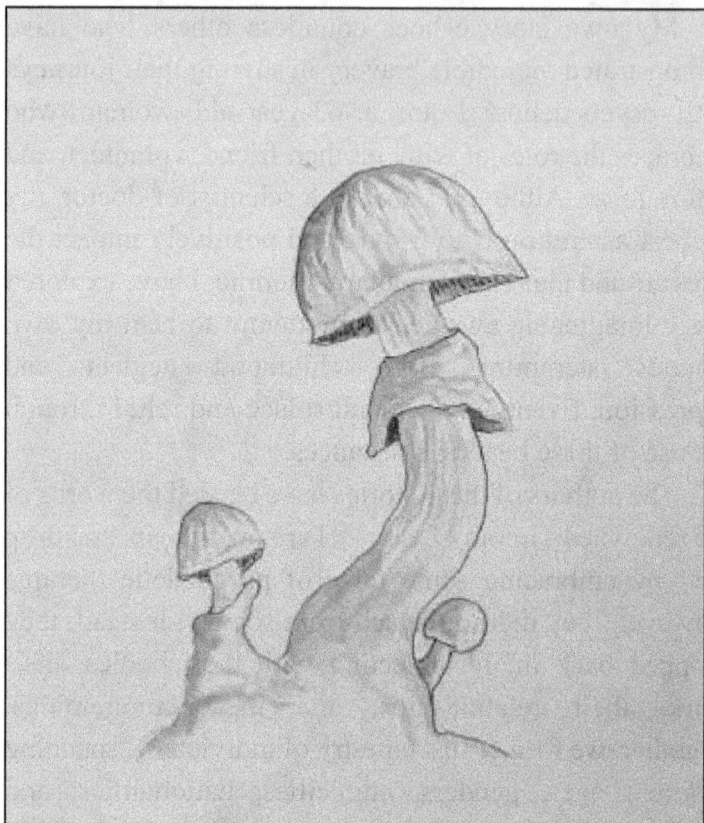

STORIES OF HEALING
EXPERIENCES WITH PLANT
MEDICINE
Psilocybin

Psilocybin is a naturally occurring psychedelic compound found in over 200 species of fungi. It's typically ingested via fresh or dried mushrooms, tea made from dried mushrooms, or capsules. The liver converts psilocybin into psilocin upon ingestion, which results in changes in perception, mood, and consciousness. Psilocybin has been used for religious and spiritual practices in various cultures for thousands of years. Since the 1960s, clinical trials have also suggested that psilocybin might be successful in treating many conditions such as depressive disorders, anxiety, substance abuse, anorexia, obesity, and cluster headaches.

In the early 60s, Timothy Leary and Richard Alpert established a series of experiments called the Harvard Psilocybin Project. Leary and Alpert believed in the therapeutic benefits of psilocybin, and conducted studies in a "naturalistic setting" as well as at Concord State Prison. Unfortunately, the project was shut down in 1962 after Leary and Alpert violated their agreement with Harvard by administering psilocybin to an undergraduate.

In 1962, Walter Panke conducted his Good Friday– or Marsh Chapel–experiment to demonstrate how psychedelics mimic life-changing, mystical experiences. Panke's study was conducted on divinity students who voluntarily took part in his experiment. In 1986, Rick Doblin of MAPS interviewed all but one of the divinity students from the Marsh Chapel experiment. Most had reported that the experience had profoundly reshaped their lives and it continued all those years later. Doblin's findings are consistent with typical accounts of psilocybin use, as many individuals have reported still experiencing benefits 10-20 years after psilocybin use, such as a sense of compassion, gratitude, peace, and belonging.

By 1968, the possession of psychedelics was criminalized in the U.S. under the Staggers-Dodd Bill. Medical and scientific research on psilocybin was brought to a full halt in 1971 after President Richard Nixon declared the "War on Drugs." Today, many organizations are focused on psychedelic research such as the Multidisciplinary Association for Psychedelic Studies (MAPS), numerous clinical trials and major universities worldwide.

PSILOCYBIN STORIES

Male / 40 / Texas / Rancher

Smoked for 25 years. Got to be 3 packs a day. Doctor gave me a death sentence if I didn't stop. Wife gave me an ultimatum. Son and friends used mushrooms occasionally for entertainment. They also knew if used in a therapeutic setting, it was supposed to stop addictions. Not really my style but they helped find me a 'guide' to help with the therapeutic part. We talked a couple of times before. Then we met on the day of the 'event'. I am a bit embarrassed to say but I was scared as hell. Since I have never done anything other than a beer or two. Letting go was very hard for me. He said it would start hitting me in about 30 minutes but it took almost 90 because I was resisting. Since nothing was happening with my resistance, I guess I relaxed and it started working. All I can say is that it was the most beautiful experience of my life. I had never felt so much love, compassion and acceptance. By the next day I had this sudden desire to take care of myself in so many ways. Not only did I feel valuable and blessed, I felt an urge to take care of what I had. Smoking turned my stomach when the automatic pilot set in to grab a cigarette and light it. I felt a sense to slow down and take in the beauty around me. The junk food I was also addicted to no longer called my name.

It's been about 5 months now and I haven't had a smoke. For some reason an apple or orange sounds so much better than Fritos or cupcakes. Don't really understand how it worked but it did.

Female / 32 / San Jose, CA / Accountant

My healing journey these past couple of years has been with Ketamine with myself and my therapist. I recently had an amazing opportunity to participate in a psilocybin women's weekend retreat with five other women who are also on this healing path.

Though I was nervous and didn't know the other participants very well, I left the weekend experience with a new found longing to expand my healing practice in an extroverted way. I left with a desire to search for more events where I can be with others in this special headspace, to volunteer and give back to the community, to help it continue to flourish; possibly through my career path and finance skills.

I had only consumed psilocybin a handful of times before but the wisdom received from my dedicated Ketamine practice, and the loving support I received from multiple systems allowed me to sink into and set an intention of "be open, and allow".

My journey began the moment I decided to participate in this retreat. I spent many weeks preparing, with a special focus the two days before. My preparation included a healthy diet, yoga, meditation, a therapy session, taking a day off of work, and relying on my partner for support so I could focus on myself.

The medicine space on that day was very kind. I couldn't stop smiling and feeling deep gratitude for so many things including the women I was with, the space that was held for us, for being alive at this time in history, for the generations before me who protected and passed on this wisdom... I also experienced a special connection with my inner goddess, which was reflected back to me by the facilitators in a beautiful way that caused an unexpected emotional reaction which was very cathartic.

The integration has been deep and meaningful. I'm finding myself choosing healthier meals and habits, avoiding the news, and a general slowing down. I feel more connected to all women I think of or come in contact with.

I would recommend group medicine healing for anyone and everyone on this path. I was reminded that many traditional healing experiences took place in group, tribal settings around a fire with multiple generations. There is something uniquely special and impactful about being vulnerable in a group, being a witness and being witnessed, and feeling seen and validated by a group of likeminded souls.

Female / 61 / Southern CA / Retired

After doing several sessions with a psychedelic integration coach we met for the big day. I ate the dried mushrooms, sat in the sun for about 15 minutes then it started. I was very nervous as I hadn't really done any 'drugs' before. She had me lay down, cover my eyes and played some music. The 'medicine' came on slowly. At first it was just some beautiful colors and designs. Then it started getting a little scary because everything would go dark with each heartbeat. I was concerned it would stay dark but it didn't. There was a huge abundance of information being shown to me. Like watching a movie. Things I was shown seemed to be from a higher source, things I had forgotten. Things I knew in my brain but not my heart and the information reached my heart. But not in an emotional way. In a matter-of-fact way. My personality was never one to speak up or be the one in charge. But the information coming in was that I had a voice and I was meant to use it. People will listen, people are interested in what knowledge I have to offer. There was a lot of throat clearing and feeling of getting my throat and voice to be clear and unstuck. A lot of cleaning out if you will.

At any time, I could have stopped it all. It was kind of like a waking daydream. I didn't feel out of control and I just kept welcoming the messages coming in. Which seemed like a flood. I tried to tell my coach some of the things so she could write them down but there was just so much.

Afterwards, I was a little disappointed because everyone talks about these HUGE experiences they have. Mine was gentle and not overwhelming. But as I thought about it later when I was feeling greedy about not getting enough. The realization was that too much would have probably been way too overwhelming for me. And as days went by the quiet slow healing continued. My sense of having a voice to speak up became stronger and stronger.

I remembered who I was not who I was told I was. My belief is that the 'medicine' is intelligent and knows what you need and what you can handle if you are taking it for healing. I will probably do it again sometime within a year and maybe take a larger dose (but not a lot larger). Coaches are great because they really help integrate feelings after the session. I also journal almost every day and meditate most days.

Male / 50 / Canada / Technology

My mother passed away. She and I were very close and it was years later that I was still in a very deep depression because of grief. Someone suggested a mushroom journey to me and I thought "what do I have to lose?" This friend found me a therapist that was using mushrooms underground along with therapy. Cutting to the chase, it was amazing. I was able to reconnect with my mother on the journey and got an extreme sense that she was well where she was. As I came out of the journey, an instant feeling of weight and depression lifted and has never returned. It was what I needed to be able to become a joyful functioning man again.

Female / 38 / Ohio / Barista

For most of my life that I can remember. I had migraine headaches. Even as a kid I would get them often. I would eventually throw up and feel better. But it was like being hit by a train afterwards. As an adult, I started missing so much work I changed jobs a lot.

One day randomly, I was speaking with a friend at work. She was telling me that she had a similar problem. She told me that two years ago she was chosen for a trial with Psilocybin for migraines. And that she hasn't had a migraine since! I was all in at that point. The problem was the legality of getting some and there weren't any trials where I lived. Much to my outright joy, she was able to get some mushrooms for me from a friend of a friend sort of thing. She offered to sit with me and tried to do a copy of what the trial had done with her. Talking about my intentions beforehand. She also gave me an idea of what to expect during the trip. We set up my living room for the big day. She downloaded a playlist for me to listen to and got me a cozy mask to wear to cover my eyes. Under the influence of the mushrooms, it is very hard to describe but not something I ever experienced. I felt that I got a lot of love, compassion and encouragement from somewhere. When it was over about 5 hours later, I ate a little something and she left. For the next couple of weeks, she and I had a lot of discussions to debrief regarding the trip. Which was so helpful because she understood what it was like. She also found me an online zoom community to keep integrating.

What I was shown is that I hold tight to all of my stress. That it isn't necessary. -a surprisingly simple message. I listened and am now doing what some people might think is weird but works for me. Like screaming into pillows or jumping up and down when I am feeling stress. I have had some light headaches but nothing at all like a migraine. It has changed me and my life. What a gift she gave me!!!! I would be willing to do it again to get rid of all headaches. Which I may when the time and opportunity appear.

Male / 57 / Umbria Italy / Train Operator

I met a man from Australia. During a short conversation that went deep quickly he told me about his recent experience with (as you in the USA call them) magic mushrooms. It was something I knew nothing about but it really attracted my interest. I spent many months researching what these plants could do for my personal healing.

As it turns out, there are a lot of people using them in my area so it wasn't too difficult to find a teacher to help me with the process.

I know this is anonymous but I don't feel comfortable writing about my problems. What I will tell you is that after 3 sessions and talking with my teacher regularly I am remarkably better. My brain works so much better. My emotions are under control and I am comfortable being the man I am.

Female / 50 / Northern CA / Counselor

I suffered from Fibromyalgia and severe PMS. After trying many mainstream prescriptions and finding no relief, someone suggested mushrooms. In my desperation of feeling so terrible for so long, I took the leap. Since I live in northern CA, Oakland is a town where it is easier to access them. It is also very easy to find a trained underground guide in my area when I got the courage to ask around. After one large dose and a LOT of emotional release all day, it was a miracle how much better my health was. It is unbelievable how our body deteriorates holding onto all the crap. I have decided to continue microdosing and am seeing slow and steady progress in continual healing. No more prescriptions for me!

Male / 55 / Australia / Engineer

Watching my father struggle with Cancer and his devastating decline was so wrenching to witness. In the thick of this dying process that he was kicking and resisting the whole way, a doctor recommended a psilocybin journey. I was shocked, but he consented. After that journey, he was a whole new person. He relaxed into his illness and imminent death. It made such a difference for the whole family and him in letting him go into a peaceful death. It seemed to take away his fear and resistance to the eventual situation. I am considering doing a journey myself now.

Female / 62 / Northern CA / Yoga Instructor

Healing depression with these medicines. This journey was mushrooms paired with MDMA. This is how I described my journey in my writing circle 2 days later.
"Don't forget to be human," she said. "Oh honey, let me show you what it is to be loved". She took me. Filled me. Showed me. Then she dissolved me and showed me the whole of it, the LOVE, the whole universe of dark and

stars and aching beauty, but it didn't ache. It WONDERED! It was WONDER. It was the whole of everything and it was, what? God? Love? She just kept showing me: this is love, it's all love, you are love, you can't help it, you just are. Nothing for it, just love. We all are, we come from it and return to it and in the meantime we are placed into human bodies to….what? You see. I have made a lifetime out of not being, crafting and perfecting my project of becoming smaller and paler and lighter, of disappearing, like that could quell the astonishingly loud experience of this being human. It all just FELT like too much. It scared me, all this feeling. "Don't forget to be human," she said as she delivered me back to earth. "Land hard right here in this gift you have been given. Even your pain is exquisite and you've had the gift of that!" All the words I'd heard and read and steeped in and tried so very hard to understand, I now understood in an instant. In that experience, in that place she showed me, it all became so simple and clear. Since then, it's gotten cloudy again but I'm working hard to remember.

Female / 73 / Ontario / Retired Therapist

My whole life I just felt like I was trying. Trying to please, trying to prove, trying to earn my keep, trying not to take up too much space. At 70, I just got sick and tired of all the trying and it never being enough. By chance I ran into an old friend. We had coffee and she had just had this amazing experience with mushrooms she told me. She couldn't say enough about how it has and is changing her life. Since I always feel these types of things happened for a reason and the right time, I asked for her assistance to do what she experienced.

Two weeks later, I was speaking with her Psychedelic Integration Coach. We had several sessions so she could get to know me, what my life was like and what my intentions were in doing this work. A month after that was my big day. Of course I was nervous. Even though I was around all the psychedelics in my youth, it wasn't something I had ever done.

The experience is so hard to put into words. Saying that it was the most beautiful, wonderful experience of my life doesn't even cover it. The medicine showed me that I was so loved, so beautiful, so important, so valuable it makes me cry even writing this. All the trying was so very unnecessary. I am amazing just because I am a child of God put on this earth. Other humans have their own issues and try to make us feel lesser than. But none of us are lesser than another. It's so interesting how we all forget all that when we come to earth.

I still speak with my coach because as a retired therapist I know integration is so important. I journal, pray and exercise daily to take care of myself. I was given the gift of life and want to honor that by taking care of me. Which also in turn helps me take care of others better. I wish I would have known about this during my career. How much more helpful could I have been to my patients

Female / 46 / Portland, OR / Social Worker

January of 2018 at the age of 40, I found myself pondering where I had been, where I was, and where to go from here. Divorced with six kids, working multiple jobs for barely a living wage as a social worker, and scraping to make ends meet, I decided it was time to reach inward. I started by attending a co-dependency anonymous group where I began a 12-step program by writing and reading my life story in all its gore and glory to a room of strangers.

A woman in the group began to cry saying she felt traumatized by my story. I was at a loss for a response. Luckily, two people came to my rescue. They explained to her that the process of healing begins with laying all of our cards out on the table in a safe environment where we can support one another and work through what haunts us, and what keeps us trapped in unhealthy patterns. And so, my journey into the depths of self-discovery took on a new chapter.

I became a relentless seeker with a hyper-focus on the big questions…who am I? Why am I? What am I here for? Where was I before I was here and where will I be when it's time for my body to die? And how did it all come to be? The thing that bonded Jim (a new friend from that group) and I most was our unwavering love of God, or what we felt towards the concept of God as too big to describe in words. What we wanted to investigate was who, why, what, where and how is God?

I wrapped myself in a hand-made crocheted blanket created by my great-grandma when I was just a baby. I swiftly gulped down the cool brew, bits and all. I was pleasantly surprised that it did not cause any sort of stomach upset. I sat back, closed my eyes and began breathing with intention taking double inhales, holding my breath for a few seconds and slowly exhaling until I felt at ease. Slowly, a sound began to grow that eventually filled the room. It was low and deep. A vibration that conjured up visions of roots, rich dark soil, a grounded and gravitational pull that put my soul at ease. The beating like a heart became fuller until the sounds of a thousand drums hummed in a heavy tone that took me home. In a moment of recognition, I lifted my head as if to look up at last to say hello back to whatever this was. I felt an energy that was distinctly separate from me, and yet, it was coming from inside of me. As I lifted my face and opened my embrace, the sound went up too! The most soft and profound melody continued to fill the room! It was as if the sound of a thousand angels appeared! Tears streamed down my face as this sound folded me into its presence. I realized I was interacting with it, as if "it" was an "it" at all! That word seems an insult, yet I was in awe of its nature apart and yet, a part of me. I played with this sound, whichever way I went, in or out, up or down, it followed me. I was leading "it" in an orchestra of the most majestic music I have ever encountered, multiplied by infinity! After a while, I thought, if this is not just me, and it's something beyond me, maybe it has known more than me and I can ask it a question. My mind immediately went to my oldest son whose suffering weighed heavy on my heart since what feels like forever. I directed my confusion and frustration about this situation towards the sound. It replied with a goodbye, not in any kind of mean or rejection sort of way, but in a way that said, "save that for another day." It slowly drifted up and away like a breeze blowing a balloon into the distant sky. I thought, "oh, okay, bye!" and then just like the scene from Wizard of Oz when Dorothy's house abruptly lands and she walks in utter silence through the door, so did I.

I spent several weeks in bewildered contemplation of my introduction to this marvelous plant medicine. It was changing me in such subtle, yet profound ways. I sang throughout the day and especially in the shower! My walk became more relaxed. I was extra focused at work and present with my family. I noticed and appreciated the things that I took for granted before; sunsets, birds, the wind, and especially moving water. I had started attending an ecstatic dance event every Sunday morning which I called "church" and I noticed that my dance was changing too. I felt more in my body and less in worry about how I appeared to others. I danced often with my eyes closed, spinning in circles like a whirling dervish, imagining the holy spirit in form as he had appeared in a dream in the weeks before as both an old wise man on my left and a small child to my right. Together, we flowed, effortlessly!

The next time, I took the mushrooms, I pulled a blanket over my body and took deep breaths, reminding myself that the only way out was through. I knew I was safe and not at risk of causing myself any harm. The medicine would know what I needed. I let go and allowed the mushrooms to take the wheel. There was a deep sound as tears streamed down my face. The tears did not come from fear or pain, nor was it sadness, despair, shame, remorse, or even joy. It was a feeling that to this day I cannot find a word to describe. It just was. These intense sensations went on for some time until all at once, the experience slowed to a full stop. I sat upright on the edge of the bed as if sitting on the edge of a swimming pool that I had just emerged from. I wiped the tears and snot from my face, took a deep breath and looked around. Immediately, a tidal wave of emotion came flying at me, hitting me hard enough to cause a whole new flood of tears, shaking me to my very soul. This time I recognized it, it was gratitude. An overwhelming feeling that I had everything I needed came over me. Nothing was missing, broken, lacking or lost. Everything was perfectly in place, as it should be, as it would be, as it had always been.

Female / 74 / Undisclosed / Retired professional

A lot of people around me did psychedelics in my youth, but not me. As a typical woman I learned to put everyone above me. As I reached menopause, I grew more and more depressed. Therapy didn't work. SSRIs didn't work. Running into a very old friend was my saving grace. She shared her experience with healing with psychedelics and talked me into giving it a try with her coach. I was excited, very nervous, curious and hopeful. This is what happened; the medicine let me connect with my own inner wisdom that I had long pushed aside. It gave me permission to do what I need, what I want to do, to put myself first instead to become happy again. And by

God, it is working. At first, I didn't even know what I needed or wanted. It had been so many years since I even considered those subjects. But after giving myself permission, it was steady slow progress but it is working. My joy in life is returning. I am learning who I am for the first time in my adult life. It is an experience that I would continue doing to heal. Lots of paying attention, integration, journaling and meditation but it is really worth it.

Female / 52 / Northern California / Workforce Trainer

I was determined to heal before I lost everything. A diagnosis of complex PTSD was a complete relief because I finally found out what was wrong with me (high anxiety, loss of learning ability, feelings of helplessness, and lots of frustration). But talk therapy and EMDR treatment wasn't dislodging the emotions that were stuck and most of the time I felt dead inside. I'd never taken any drugs when young, except for a bit of recreational pot, so I was nervous. Not only was it illegal, I had no idea what it would do. I ordered spores and grew my own mushrooms while studying the research and reading "How to Change Your Mind". Then I eased into it, a very small dose, then double that, but wasn't feeling anything but relaxation. Finally, I decided to try a larger dose, in a friend's backyard under his watchful eye for safety.

About an hour in, I swirled into the sky as a spiral of glittering dust, then marveled at the growing grass and trees. It was easy to see we were all the same, all vibrantly energetic and I could see that energy. The most important realization was that I could remember who I really was, a soul visiting earth as a human, and that most of the time I was in a dream state. Except on mushrooms. Then I was awake and able to remember so clearly that not only was I incredibly strong, but that there were many other souls helping me out, and cheering me on. I asked if I could study this science of spirituality and a voice came back: "We want you to." Then I started thinking of the lost souls in the world, the other souls who were in so much pain and I wept and wept for us all, then a sudden silence and the most profound stillness I could imagine, as if I'd been given the gift of a long break from my always overactive and anxious mind. Time stopped. Squirrels and birds came close, and I stood holding a tree branch in silence and peace. There was later a wave of gratitude and incredible love, it was as if I was being healed by it. I remember about this time asking how long I'd been under this and my friend replied 3 hours. Then I was grateful I had another 3 or so hours to enjoy that feeling of love.

It took less of a dose to feel this way a few months later. I was thinking of my deceased mother when I consumed them. I was shown a door with a seam of intensely bright and beautiful light around its edges. I knew I was supposed to open doors, go up or down stairs, etc., because these are common themes in other people's journeys. But I was feeling "chicken" and so I explained I was too afraid to open the door and go through. And so, the door opened anyway and my mother came out. She

27

looked like mostly light, but I could recognize her. She didn't speak, only stayed with me sharing incredible love.

After another medium dose several months later, I again felt that feeling of waking up from the dream and knowing who I really was, and I felt like life was too intense, too hard, too painful. And as soon as I realized I was with my guides, my deeply loving friends, I asked why it was so incredibly hard to live on earth and was told it was important that I be here for learning. And the large group told me I was doing very well, and they came close around me in a tight and loving circle of protection, telling me I could reach them whenever I wanted.

Since, in my profession, I am an expert in learning and development, and have written a book on workforce training, the pieces came together and I know this whole experience was a training program. And that lessons were repeated until we learned them, and that the goal is to evolve our soul so that we do not get stuck in negative emotions while experiencing life on a beautiful blue planet stocked with everything we need. The sad times aren't meant to last forever, and letting go was one of my hardest but most beneficial lessons. Now I meditate to simply feel that circle of love around me, and occasionally doing a small dose is enough to get me centered, connected and relaxed and able to see what emotions I might have stored somewhere in the body that needs to be let go.

Male / 64 /Alabama / Consultant

(As reported over the phone)

At the age of 60, Robert stood at a pivotal juncture in his life, burdened by a sense of stagnation and unrealized dreams. Determined to find a fresh perspective, he embarked on a transformative psilocybin journey guided by experienced facilitators in the tranquil embrace of nature. As the mystical effects of the psilocybin unfurled, Robert's consciousness expanded, dissolving the confines of his perception. In this altered state, he was confronted with the raw truths of his fears and regrets, but also with the dormant reservoir of untapped potential residing within him.

Immersed in a swirling kaleidoscope of vibrant colors and intricate patterns, Robert encountered profound insights and a flood of long-suppressed emotions. The protective walls he had constructed around his heart began to crumble, and he was bathed in a profound sense of self-compassion and acceptance. With each breath, he released the weight of past mistakes and embraced a newfound appreciation for the preciousness of the present moment. The healing power of the psilocybin journey liberated Robert from the chains of self-doubt, empowering him to embark on a courageous voyage of self-discovery. Fueled by a renewed zest for life, he vowed to pursue his passions with unwavering determination, ultimately rewriting the narrative of his life's final chapter.

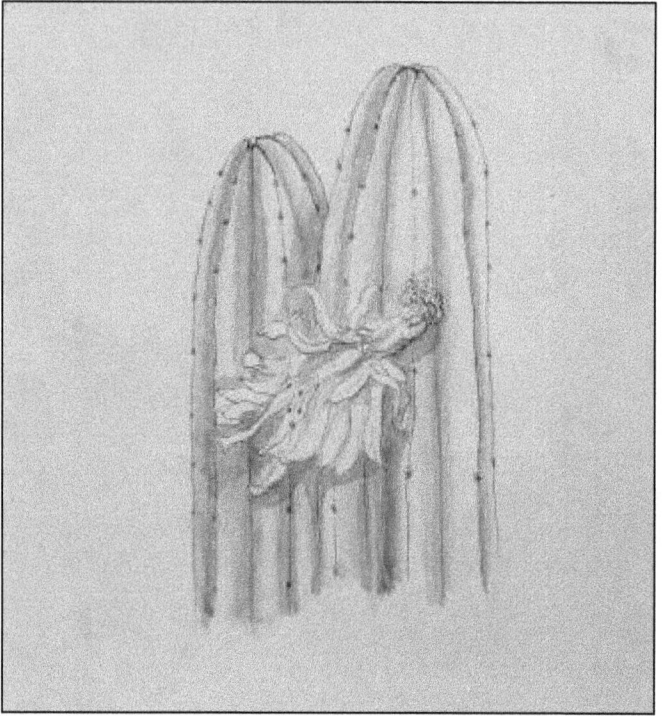

STORIES OF HEALING
EXPERIENCES WITH PLANT
MEDICINE
Mescaline (Huachuma)

Mescaline, a naturally occurring psychedelic compound, is found in several cacti, most notably the San Pedro (*Echinopsis pachanoi*) and the spineless peyote (*Lophophora williamsii*). Mescaline is typically consumed orally as a tea. It has been used for many generations and has played a role in Indigenous religious ceremonies in North America for over five thousand years.

Research indicates that mescaline, when combined with therapy, may be effective in treating addiction to alcohol and other substances. It has also shown potential for alleviating anxiety and depression.

In the United States, mescaline is classified as a Schedule I substance under the Controlled Substances Act, making its use illegal for recreational or therapeutic purposes outside of specially approved research settings. However, exemptions exist for certain Indigenous communities, where the use of mescaline is permitted as part of traditional religious practices.

Peyote, which grows naturally in limited regions of the southern United States and Mexico, faces significant challenges to its survival. The species is in decline due to several factors. Increased demand, a growing number of non-Indigenous users seek to experience peyote, putting pressure on its natural supply. Habitat loss because of cattle ranching, agriculture, and oil and gas development have encroached on the desert landscapes where peyote thrives. Overharvesting, poaching and unsustainable harvesting practices have decimated wild populations.

Adding to these challenges, peyote is a slow-growing plant, taking a decade or more for a seed to develop into a mature cactus with sufficient mescaline for consumption. As a result, peyote is now considered a vulnerable species, prompting calls for more responsible use and conservation.

For many Indigenous peoples, peyote holds profound spiritual and ceremonial significance. Within the Native American Church (NAC), it is considered sacred, used in rituals to promote healing, guidance, and connection to the divine. Members of the NAC have urged non-Indigenous people to abstain from harvesting or using peyote out of respect for its cultural importance and to ensure its preservation.

To address this scarcity, some suggest turning to alternative sources of mescaline, such as the more abundant San Pedro cactus, which grows faster and does not share the same vulnerability status as peyote. This shift helps protect peyote while still allowing individuals to explore mescaline's effects in a sustainable and culturally sensitive manner.

MESCALINE STORIES

Male / 67 / Boston, MA / Sports Industry

After witnessing a few athletes successfully use this type of therapy, I decided to try it myself. Throughout my life, I struggled with severe negativity—especially towards myself, but also towards everything and everyone around me. As much as I hate to admit it, it was utterly exhausting. After studying how this therapy could fundamentally change the way the brain operates, I decided to give it a shot.

During the first ceremony I attended, I realized that we are all connected. I learned that by criticizing a stranger, I was ultimately hurting myself. In the second ceremony, I discovered that I am deeply loved and valuable. I understood that I am an important part of humanity and that what I say and think matters profoundly. The third ceremony was so complex that I can't even begin to describe it in words, but I can tell you that I emerged as a changed human being. This transformation has positively affected not only me but also those around me.

Male / 54 / Ashland, OR / Massage Therapist

As an alternative healing practitioner, I spend my time searching for natural healing methods. My life experiences have left me with scars that with all my knowledge still wasn't healing. This is one of those friend of a friend situations. A friend knew a guy who did healing with San Pedro ceremonies. It was local to me and the ceremony date fit into my schedule. No brainer. I can take a hint from the universe.

This medicine gently knocked my socks off. It was an all-night affair with sacred fire and filled with intention. By the next morning my body and brain were buzzing with such an overwhelming sense of love and belonging. It's so very hard to describe in words. The bottom line is that I was lacking those two things and didn't even realize it. SP gave me that. With both of those feelings, it is so much easier now for me to do the work to continue to heal. Note that I AM DOING THE WORK. SP doesn't just magically heal. It helps us to do the work more successfully.

Male / 50 / Washington / Business owner

I really tried everything. Self-help books, yoga, listening to podcasts, you name it. I once heard someone say when they pray for patience, they get traffic. -That was me. When it seemed I could do it myself, I was shown time and time again that I couldn't. Then one day, I was listening to Joe Rogan on YouTube. He was interviewing Michael Pollan and they were talking about peyote. It hit me, that's what I needed to try. But since peyote is an endangered plant, I decided to find someone who would work with me with San Pedro. I found a great guy in Oregon who had his own cactus farm, was a coach and very knowledgeable about SP. He was the most kind and gentle huge teddy bear of a guy. Honestly, I was nervous as hell but he really made me feel comfortable enough to relax and let the medicine do its thing. These plants are said to have wisdom and now I am a believer. I went in with intentions but the plant 'knew' exactly what I needed. It showed me, there is no reason to be impatient for anything. Time is forever, so why the rush. The weird thing is that I actually FELT that. It wasn't like someone telling you something and you don't really believe it. It showed me that things get done, completed, go on as they should without my help. My angst won't help anything. It is really difficult to find convincing words to tell my story yet I know it is true for me. Reasons I am sure scientists have studied but I can't explain. My brain seems to have changed. I have gone back to my coach now three times over the years and each time, I am shown something new and amazing. Which helps me to be a better person. If we all could become a better form of ourselves, wouldn't this world be an amazing place?

Female / 65 / Laguna Beach, CA / Shop Owner

I have always been into natural medicine and healing. When I started feeling the middle life blues of what next, I started talking to a lot of women my age. One day an acquaintance invited me to meet her 'guide' who she had been working with for several years. His specialty is in San Pedro therapy. We really hit it off and although I didn't feel like I had a lot to 'fix' just some decisions to make and to shake the blues off, I decided to start meeting with him.

He was very careful to start at a lower dose and see how I responded. It almost didn't seem like much was happening. I seemed completely coherent, could have got up to use the restroom or get a drink if I had wanted. Yet I was getting some sort of wisdom download. Quiet revelations and suggestions. Things that I wasn't consciously aware of. There was an acute awareness also. I thought I was relaxed yet I kept being shown areas in my body that weren't really. I would loosen up those areas just to be shown another. Or the same areas again and again as the tightness crept back in. Even my scalp seemed a bit tight. It made me realize that although my interpretation was of being relaxed, I was not. This went on for several hours and was quite pleasant. All I had to do was pay attention and relax the parts when I noticed. It was very interesting because by relaxing those parts, it seemed to let something release each time. I don't know exactly what but apparently it was something I have been holding onto quite tightly.

After it seemed like it was over, my guide gave me some tea and a snack. I felt completely normal, just 100% more relaxed and lighter than after the best massage you could ever imagine. We talked for a while but I couldn't explain what I released. He said that it doesn't matter. Sometimes it's not even explainable. It just is. It's strange because now I seem to be out of the blues and ready for the next stage of my life. Whatever I was holding onto seems to have released the blue mood I was feeling. This was so much healthier than going on medication and it was easy. Not at all what I expected.

Female / 71 / Medford, OR / Retired Dentist

This may sound a little flippant but I have done a lot of psychedelics in my life. Almost all for entertainment until the last 5 years. When I started hearing that these substances can be healing if used in an intentional way, I started reading volumes. It had never occurred to me to take psychedelics and heal. I took them and sat in nature to watch the trees or at a party to have fun dancing and mingling. Now that I am getting older and things are catching up with me; regrets, wasted time, aches and pains…my opinion has changed about how they should be used. Ok, jumping off my soapbox now.

It was easy to find someone to help me use San Pedro as a healing medicine. People have been doing it for centuries. Referred to often as the grandfather medicine. Out of all the substances, it is the most gentle in my opinion. I started talking to this medicine man as a therapist. He isn't a licensed therapist but is probably much better considering he is a 7th generation medicine man working with Huachuma. We talked about all the things I did, regret but can't change. About my future intention of taking care of my body and forgiving myself for said regrets. Talking was the majority of my healing. Sometimes with San Pedro and sometimes without. It was an ongoing process of about 6 months, all the while journaling to keep track of emotions, physical feelings, thoughts etc.

Fast forward to now; I am feeling amazing. I have forgiven myself for a lot of mistakes, asked others still around to forgive me, have made progress actually LOVING myself and being comfortable with who I am. A lot of my physical pains have dissipated. Probably because my mood is better and I am taking much better care of myself. Why didn't I know about this aspect of these substances earlier in my life? Probably because there is such a stigma around using them for any reason. I pray that changes, because it can help a lot of lives.

Male / 29 / Santa Fe, NM / Restaurant Owner

San Pedro is a garden plant where I live. It's legal until you process it. For many many generations people around my hometown have used it for ceremonies. It was and is for religious and social purposes with many people groups. If tribes were not getting along, they would gather and do ceremonies together and work things out peacefully. It is used for healing many different ailments as a medicine. So, when I felt like I needed to heal my heart from life that is what I turned to. I just felt like my heart had hardened to stone. I didn't care and knew I should.

It was easy to find a shaman in my area to assist me. We met for a while to get to know each other and so he could understand why I wanted help. The culture treats this plant with complete reverence. They want to protect traditions with the utmost care and honor.

When I went in for my ceremony there was a beautiful altar. It had feathers, stones and many other objects from nature. I bought some items with meaning for me to add. The shaman sang some beautiful significant songs, said a prayer to the different directions, north, west, south and east. He asked for protection from the ancestors for both he and I. It was a beautiful ceremony before the medicine ceremony. Then I drank the tea made from the cactus. After an hour, I drank a little more. It seemed a little hard for me to let go so a while later, a third cup.

Then it all started. The more I relaxed and let go, the more I was shown. I just had to trust the wisdom to gain the knowledge it could give me. There was so much and it would sound crazy if I told the details. The underlying and most important message was that it's all love. EVERYTHING. Nothing else matters. Love for our ancestors, love for our planet, love for ourselves and love for each other. My heart was pulsating with a green light. This greenlight was just blasting into it from the universe. It felt like it was healing every cell of my heart and softening the stone it had become. Tears fell and didn't stop. I was so grateful. Grateful for everything. That was the second message I received; be grateful for EVERYTHING.

And today years later, I still hold and feel those lessons. My heart is open and what an amazing feeling that is.

Male / 22 / World Citizen / Adventure Seeker

I've been spending a lot of time in South America rock climbing, and down here, San Pedro is just a normal conversation. It's also legal, so it's pretty easy to find a ceremony with people who really know what they're doing. That's one of the best parts—getting to learn from locals who treat the medicine with respect. But there's also a downside. A lot of psychedelic tourism is sketchy, and it doesn't feel right to me.

Back home in Appalachia, things were rough. My house was pretty messed up, and by 15, I'd had enough. I took off to figure myself out and have some kind of adventure. Peru was my first stop—cheap to live, and I had a friend who traded me a flight in exchange for teaching her to rock climb. After that, I just kept moving around, meeting amazing people, and learning about life.

When I found out about San Pedro, I was curious, but I didn't expect how much it would change me. I started doing ceremonies with locals, and it's been healing in ways I can barely explain. All the anger I had toward certain people, the worthlessness I carried—it's mostly gone. The medicine helped me see that I'm loved and valuable, that I've always had something to give the world. It wasn't me who was broken; it was my circumstances.

I'm so grateful I ended up here because it's made me a better person—completely different from who I was when I left. I'll go back to the States someday, but not until I feel like I've finished this work on myself. Back where I'm from people never heard of doing this kind of healing.

Female / 62 / Oregon / Tour Planner

I have never been one to do drugs but I met someone at a biohacking conference I was attending. He was talking about San Pedro and what a wonderful healing plant it was. I had been feeling really low for a while but didn't think much about doing that sort of thing. A couple of months went by and things just lined up for an opportunity to try San Pedro in a small group setting. It was one of those things that a bunch of things happen that just give you a nudge through the door. So, I went. I was one of the older people there. The leader and his wife were my age, the rest were many years younger. Since it was all new to me, I took the smallest dose (one cup of tea) but after 90 minutes, feeling the same, I had a 2nd. I didn't feel like I was affected except I was shaking and my head started hurting but not like a headache. Like something was trying to release. When I told our leader/healer he gave me a head massage and blew ceremonial tobacco on my head and something did release in a big way. After that when the group was going around the circle at the sacred fire and talking one at a time. It was very strange but all of these very wise things came out of my mouth in support of each of the younger members of the group. It seemed to really make a difference in their experience.

Would I do it again? Probably yes and I would drink a little more tea. I felt like there was quite a bit of trauma released from my body during that experience. But it seemed that San Pedro was using me as a helper for the group that night. I didn't mind helping others in their healing. Isn't that why we are all here anyways? To support each other.

Female / 50 / New Jersey / Neurologist

Since I am a doctor of the brain and a scientist at heart, I did extensive research on several of these healing medicines. I kept hearing such amazing stories of healing. I decided I was going to grow my own San Pedro plants just to have a relationship with the plants. Just growing them, I realized how sacred they are. When the opportunity came up it appeared it was time for me to take a journey myself. It was with a Shaman that was working with these plants for many years.

The experience was beautiful, loving and eye opening. It was love, pure love. Love for myself, love for others, love for the beautiful planet we are all citizens of. A very kind and gentle experience. Life changing. I wanted to be part of this community. In a way, I felt very greedy. It left me wanting more, much more. But, as instructed by the Shaman, "Do the work on yourself, don't rely on just the plant doing everything for you." It

43

took almost two years of integration, and doing the work with daily revelations from the experience. Patience is what I learned and partnership with the plants. We MUST respect these intelligent plants to guide us in partnership. We MUST respect our planet where all these healing plants are growing. We MUST stop the raping of the land. The more we destroy nature, the sicker we become.

This will forever be part of my life in one way or another. People are shocked when they find out. Me, a respected doctor, doing plant medicine. So, I keep it pretty private unless I feel the need to share the information with someone. Pretty soon, hopefully, we can all share when it does not have such a stigma. San Pedro is legal in some places but still not accepted in mainstream society. One day, my friends. One day….

Male / 67 / Montana / Retired Military

Living in Montana, I have a lot of Indigenous friends. One night while drinking a few beers on one of those friends' porch, he told me about a ceremony that his family was doing that weekend. When I showed interest, but I knew nothing about that, he invited me to be a part of it. Since he was a good buddy of mine, I thought, "what the hell, this gives me a chance to know more about his people and heritage". Well, all I can say is that it knocked my boots off! During the ceremony, I had these incredible visions of nature and how we abuse it. I am an avid hunter, mostly for sport but we don't waste the food I shoot. It never dawned on me the pain I caused the animals sometimes. In a vision, I was hunting deer. I got a shot of a beautiful female (who, in the vision, didn't realize it was female). The shot took her down and shortly after that a young calf appeared and cozied up to the mother. I felt the confusion, shock and fear of the calf. It was terrible. I had absolutely no idea of the pain my 'hobby' was causing life on our planet. After that ceremony, I never wanted to hunt again. Fishing for me from now on. And my respect, love and care for the planet have multiplied.

Non-binary / 58 / Utah / Window Installer

My brain doesn't seem to work like a normal person. Because of this I have struggled my whole life. Two years ago, someone invited me to join them in a San Pedro ceremony. He said it may give me a glimpse into the workings of my brain. It was a very crazy out of my comfort zone thing to do. But I went anyway. It didn't turn out to be completely life changing but what it did for me was give my brain space. Instead of the automatic responses that always occurred. It gave me just a few seconds of space in my reaction. Now it seems that I am able to think, feel and then actually choose how I am going to respond. It's amazing what a gift just 2 seconds can be. This has been so helpful in my happiness level. I feel that I have control now when I felt completely out of control before.

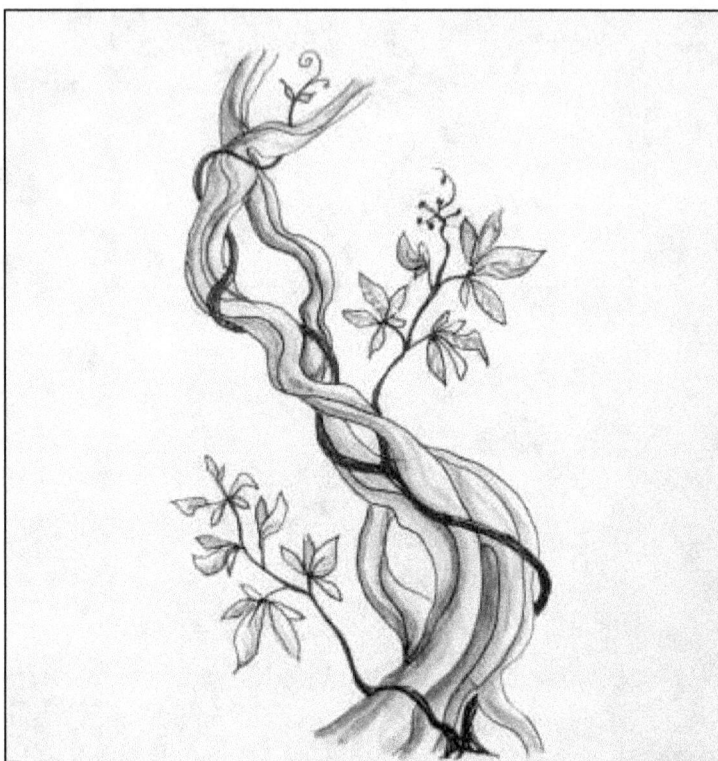

STORIES OF HEALING
EXPERIENCES WITH PLANT
MEDICINE
Ayahuasca

Ayahuasca is a potent psychedelic brew traditionally prepared from two key plants native to the Amazon basin: *Banisteriopsis caapi* (a vine) and *Psychotria viridis* (a leaf). These plants work synergistically, with *Psychotria viridis* providing DMT (N,N-dimethyltryptamine), a powerful psychoactive compound, and *Banisteriopsis caapi* acting as a monoamine oxidase inhibitor (MAOI) that prevents the digestive system from deactivating the DMT. Other plants may also be included, depending on regional traditions and the intentions of the ceremony.

Used sacramentally for over a thousand years by indigenous peoples of South America, Ayahuasca is revered for its capacity to facilitate healing, spiritual growth, and profound insight. Consumed as a tea, it often induces intense visions, physical purging, and deep emotional processing. While these effects can be challenging, they are considered integral to the transformative experience.

Ayahuasca ceremonies are typically conducted in the evening under the guidance of an experienced facilitator, often called a curandero(a) or ayahuascero. These leaders are steeped in the traditions of their lineage, using healing songs (known as *icaros*) or music to guide participants through their journeys. These songs are believed to open spiritual pathways, provide healing, and enhance individual experiences.

In preparation for the ceremony, participants are advised to follow a strict regimen to cleanse the body and mind. This often includes abstaining from substances such as alcohol, drugs, caffeine, and tobacco, as well as avoiding sexual activity, for at least a month prior. Many facilitators also recommend adhering to a vegetarian or vegan diet for 2–4 weeks beforehand to reduce toxins and promote clarity.

Research into Ayahuasca's therapeutic benefits has shown promise in areas like substance dependence, PTSD, and depression.[2] In a ceremonial or therapeutic setting, it can help individuals access and process repressed memories, facilitating deep emotional release and healing. For many, the experience provides profound spiritual guidance, insight into personal challenges, and a sense of connection to the larger universe.

While Ayahuasca remains restricted in most of the United States, it is legally consumed in certain religious contexts, such as within the *União do Vegetal* (UDV) and *Santo Daime* churches. Many seekers also travel to South America to participate in ceremonies conducted in traditional settings.

Ayahuasca is not without risks, and it should always be approached with respect and proper preparation. It is essential to participate in ceremonies led by experienced

---

[2] Saint Thomas, Sophie. "Can Psychedelics Treat Alcohol Use Disorder?" *Psychable*, 20 Oct. 2022, psychable.com/addiction/can-psychedelics-treat-alcohol-usedisorder.

and trustworthy facilitators who understand the brew's potency and the needs of participants. When consumed responsibly, Ayahuasca has the potential to be a transformative tool for healing and spiritual awakening.

AYAHUASCA STORIES

Male / 43 / Cairns, Australia / Stay at home father

My life was a constant state of fight, flight, or freeze. No matter how much yoga, meditation, or deep breathing I did, I could never really escape it. I'm not sure what wired my brain to function that way, but changing it seemed impossible on my own.

One day, I was at a park with my kids when I struck up a conversation with a woman who was there with hers. She mentioned that she had been in the same boat a few years back. She had joined a women's psychedelic group and learned about using ayahuasca for healing. If it helped her, why couldn't it help me? I asked for a contact to explore this path further.

Three months later, after several sessions with the shaman who led the healing ceremonies, I decided to take the plunge. The experience was an intense, cathartic meltdown. I can't even begin to describe it without sounding mad, but whatever hidden trauma was released felt dense, solid, and deeply rooted. The ayahuasca brought it to the surface from deep within my subconscious and yanked it out. I cried harder than I thought possible for what felt like hours. There was also a fair amount of yelling, hitting a pillow, and some strange dancing that my body just needed to do. By the time it was over, I was utterly exhausted—and yet, I felt as light as a feather.

The shaman advised me to start each day by writing

'morning pages'—three pages of whatever came into my head, without edits or distractions, until I hit the three page mark. I got up an hour before the family, found a private spot, and wrote. She also suggested never reading it, and possibly even burning it. I had about four follow-up sessions with her to debrief and integrate the experience.

Now, I'm a believer in the wisdom of these plants. I didn't know what I needed, but the plant did. I hesitate to call it magical, but it certainly feels that way. The way my brain used to default to fight, flight, or freeze is gone. Occasionally, I catch a glimpse of that old self trying to reemerge, but with my newfound awareness, I finally have the control I never had before. And YES, I would do it again.

Female / 55 / Las Vegas, NV / Computer Programmer

Hitting menopause was a bitch. My skin was crawling, I was gaining weight even though I was doing all the right things. I was very moody, and suddenly very discontented in how I had lived my life so far. I had lived for everyone else, except myself and the resentment was setting in. People (women) talk and the subject of Ayahuasca came up and how it helped with menopausal unrest. Well, I was immediately in. I was never a 'drug' taker but drank my share of adult beverages. This was supposed to be safe and less harmful on the body than alcohol. If it could cure my midlife blues/pains, it would be a good choice for me.

Two weeks later, I found myself meeting with a local underground medicine woman who was going to guide me through this journey. I felt her loving, caring presence right away and decided to work with her. She let me know that I didn't have to be 'fine' when I was around her. To heal, I needed to be honest with myself and not worry about 'looking good'.

The Ayahuasca journey was like nothing I have ever experienced. It was damn hard and emotionally draining. There was purging, bawling my eyes out, shaking and visions of ancestors who came to support me in this 'healing'. Healing it was. I left there exhausted, both mentally and physically but somehow full of deep wisdom of something I always knew but forgot. It has stuck with me and with the integration sessions with the medicine woman, I continue to heal even more. Most of my symptoms are gone. A lot of it had to do with what was in my thoughts. Heal the thoughts, heal the body. Now I am a super fan. This shit works if taken seriously and cautiously. As a side note, it is not addicting. When I was done with the journey my first thought was, I am NEVER doing that again. Someday I might but not because it was cool and fun. Just because the healing I received was worth it.

Female / 74 / Canada / Retired

After my husband of 55 years passed, I just couldn't get a grip. He was my everything. We didn't have any children and we were both only children. So, except for friends, I was alone. Three years went by. Joining grief groups, antidepressants, therapy…. nothing worked. I was actually considering suicide but my husband would be so very angry. Then one day a strange thing happened. I was watching a documentary on ayahuasca ceremonies for depression and grief. It planted a seed. Then very shortly after, I got in a discussion with a complete stranger who eventually led me to a shaman who was going to be conducting a ceremony. Well for a person who wanted to die, I didn't have any fear of trying something so foreign to my lifestyle.

Two weeks later and several sessions of intentions and 'therapy' I went to the ceremony. It was, how can I say it…. crazy and indescribable. BUT, during the ceremony, my beloved husband came to me. There was such a sense of peace that he was ok and he let me know that I was going to be ok. It was a peaceful journey for me. I expected vomiting and diarrhea but that never came. The intelligent plant knew exactly what my body and mind needed and could handle.

Afterwards, I continued with a coach and found a community of people with that experience. Each passing day the grief has blown away like the wind. I am ready to live the rest of my life the best I can and spread the wonderful news of this beautiful plant that can change your life.

Undisclosed / 45 / Toronto / Nurse

For years I have struggled with my sexual identity. It has caused me immense anxiety. So much so, I was having panic attacks several times a day. One day, a fellow nurse came into the locker room when I was in a total panic attack. She was so kind and later shared with me about an Ayahuasca experience she had. I had tried therapy and meds for years. Which weren't working so why not try something from nature. She introduced me to someone who was doing an ayahuasca ceremony the following month. I was connected with the coach holding the ceremony and we had several meetings before I joined in.

It wasn't a pretty journey. I expected to purge but boy did I ever. The feelings I had during the ceremony were heart wrenching. I couldn't cry hard enough or vomit violently enough until my system finally became empty and exhausted. But whatever the medicine did to get all that emotion and ugliness out of me was a miracle. There were many days of integration afterwards and my coach was a lifesaver. The feeling of relief was unbelievable. It was akin to losing 100 pounds of weight on my shoulders.

As the months went by with all the integration with my coach, community and journaling I decided it was time to stop hiding and show my true beautiful self to the world. I now identify as a man in a beautiful healthy woman's body and am proud of it. That has made my life a little harder with the judgment. But it is ok and the panic attacks have subsided as well as the fierce anxiety. Holding that all in was making me sick. And by the medicine helping me to let it all go, I am able to actually live my life, not just try to make it through the day.

Male / 47 / Colorado / Author

I kept hearing and reading about UDV, a small religious sect that uses ayahuasca legally, thanks to a 2006 ruling based on the Religious Freedom Restoration Act of 1993. After coming across several books and blogs on the healing benefits of ayahuasca when used in a respectful setting, I became intrigued. As a writer who relies heavily on my creative right brain, I was devastated when the dreaded writer's block struck out of nowhere. It felt more like a deep-rooted depression that stalled my entire life for several years.

They say that when you're ready, the medicine finds you. I don't know if it was mere coincidence that all the information I was consuming about ayahuasca seemed to converge at the same time, but it didn't matter—I sought out a local UDV chapter to learn more from the 'experts.' I was fortunate to find a group that was serious about using this entheogen, with no interest in entertainment (which wasn't what I was after anyway). I spent several months meeting with the shaman, learning more about her, myself, and this wondrous plant mix. Finally, she told me I was ready, and I truly felt prepared to accept what ayahuasca had to offer me.

The experience was everything you read about—purging, crying, visions—but all of it served a purpose. Ayahuasca seems to know exactly what each individual needs, which might sound like hocus pocus, but consider how many indigenous peoples have used it for healing over hundreds, if not thousands, of years. If it didn't work, people would have long forgotten about it.

I can tell you without a doubt, it worked for me, and I will never forget the blessing and privilege of using this medicine for healing. I continue to do the things to help the medicine stick and it is not a chore. My fourth (and hopefully next) bestseller is almost finished, and so is the depression.

Female / 58 / North Bay, CA / Medicine woman and artist

When I was deep into my ayahuasca practice, helping in circles every couple of months, I learned to see in the dark. I found this ability to be incredibly practical attempting to locate full buckets and offering bunches of toilet paper to participants. I also came to see and feel icaros and other medicine songs move through the space and land amongst us, sometimes inciting immense release, and sometimes giving succor.

The night I am remembering we were twenty-five or so people gathered in the Round House. The moon was nearly full, rising over the mountains, and becoming a glorious goddess crossing the sky throughout the night. I remember climbing into the music, moving slowly through the room as I joined in. Moving in reverence for the opportunity to be of service to the wisdom of these sacred plants. I felt filled with the grace of oneness and alignment. Alignment with myself and all beings in all places.

Female / 32 / Adelaide / Mother

I went to Peru, which wasn't the brightest idea but that was before these types of medicines were available in Australia and I was desperate. It was scary being in a foreign country with strangers doing something so big but I had been contemplating taking my life for a while. My husband encouraged me to go, so I went. In of itself, the whole thing was pretty traumatizing but in the end with a wonderful coach back home, he helped me integrate all that happened during the 3 ceremonies I did. It would have been much better to have found a coach before I jumped in head first. But hindsight is always so much wiser. This particular medicine is a knock your socks off operator. Grandmother Aya as she is reverently called and rightly so. She has so much power and should be respected. It is not something to take lightly when using Aya but with the right system it can be lifesaving as it was for me with the help of my coach. Grandmother Aya, showed me things I would rather have forgotten (and did before that). She also showed me that is why I had the troubles I felt I had. And most importantly, she showed me that I was deeply loved. By the planet, the cosmos, everything that was and is to come. That had never been something I had remotely known or felt. What a gift!!! I continue to do the work and it is amazing how much my life has changed and the joy I can actually feel now.

Female / 29 / Mississippi / Therapist

Since my profession is in healing others, I am always interested in healing myself so I can be the best at my job. A lot of information out there is talking about Ayahuasca and the healing from it. It scared me because I heard that you can lose control of your bowels, vomit profusely and maybe not remember some things. For a year, I researched, talked to people who had tried it and contemplated if it was right for me. I got my answer because a perfect opportunity came up. At that point, I felt it was time and I was ready.

It was all of the above that I was nervous about but I fully prepared with pre and post protocols that are recommended. Because of this experience I will be a better therapist. I can't recommend it because it isn't legal but I can share my story as best I can. That's the thing about these plant medicines; it is very difficult to tell about what actually went on in my head during the session. A lot of symbolism that may not make sense to anyone else. It hardly made sense to me at times. In the days after, I felt such a lightness. Like I lost 50 pounds of trauma I didn't even know I was carrying. It took quite some time to unwrap what some of that was but the bottom line is that it doesn't really matter to go over it all because it's gone.

Female / 33 / New York, NY/ Ballet Dancer

By the time you are in your 30's a dancing career is usually coming to a close. Younger women who have less wear and tear on their bodies usher out the older. This has been a tremendous struggle for me. My face is looking older, my body is tired with more aches and pains, even a few gray hairs. It's not just those things that bother me but combined with everything I have ever known (dance) is also slipping through my fingers. With all that, I could feel the darkness slipping in. A pre-mourning for what I was losing. Of course, no one around me understood because to the world 33 is young. There is so much life to experience. AND, I desperately wanted to feel that.

Some people I knew from high school were in town and they came to the ballet. Afterwards they sought me out to connect. They weren't close friends because even way back then, my entire life was dance. But I thought that was so nice that they made that connection that night with me. It meant so much more than I ever would have guessed. So much so that I started crying right in front of them. Since it was the last performance and I had two days off I took their offer to go out with them. During our evening together, the conversation turned to two of them having gone to an ayahuasca ceremony and how it had really changed their way of thinking about things. Of course, they also had their own struggles. How shallow was I to think that I was the only one.

Never in my wildest dreams would I have ever considered taking anything that wasn't what I was supposed to do to keep my body working like a well-oiled machine. But this new idea that came to light was, "well, what about my mind and emotions"? After hearing their stories, I was so ready to just do it. They warned me not to just jump in. If I wanted the full healing potential, I needed to do a whole series of things they recommended. All three of them were going back two months later to do a ceremony. So, I asked if I could join them. In the meantime, I researched, started journaling, and spoke several times to the shaman who was going to conduct the ceremony.

I was nervous but also excited to have the gift of a new perspective on life. And that is exactly what I got. The ceremony was wild and crazy but my takeaway was to feel so very loved, valued, part of everything and I don't have to earn it. It is my and everyone else's birthright. I am now looking forward to this new chapter in my life. Spending time with people that I never had the time to before. Feeling like I can relax and enjoy myself. Thank you Mother Aya, from my whole heart.

Female / 72 / New Zealand / Medical Researcher

Twenty years sober, yet plagued by depression. Whispers circulated about an illicit substance hailed for its healing properties. Despite being 70 years old and committed to abstaining from substances, I grappled with the weight of this decision. Would it compromise my sobriety? But what is life worth if it's merely a monotonous existence devoid of joy? Thus, I took the plunge, rushing in without any prior preparation. Perhaps out of desperation? The experience hit me like a tidal wave, leaving me disoriented for weeks on end.

Eventually, I sought the guidance of a therapist well versed in this substance. She possessed extensive knowledge and encouraged me to approach it again, but in a more informed manner. Although filled with trepidation, I embarked on the journey, knowing this time would be different.

I am profoundly grateful to my therapist for guiding me through my second encounter. It became evident that the key to using these plant medicines lies in respect, pure intentions, and integration. During the session, I was granted insights into the reasons behind my former reliance on alcohol and the newfound realization that it no longer held any power over me. Profound memories resurfaced, offering a profound understanding. Now, despite my many years of sobriety, the desire to drink has completely dissipated. The need is nonexistent. My only lament is not discovering this transformative experience three decades ago!

Male / 44 / Hamburg, Germany / Civil Engineer

Throughout most of my life, I have experienced persistent pain in my body, particularly in my legs and head. Although I would wake up each morning with a sense of anxiety, my sleep was peaceful, with pleasant dreams. I couldn't comprehend the cause behind this phenomenon. Despite having numerous reasons to be happy and grateful for my life, I found myself unable to embrace such emotions. It was during this time that a friend, who was planning a trip to the Amazon for an Ayahuasca experience, urged me to join him. Since I still had several weeks of vacation remaining, I decided to accompany him, hoping to explore its potential impact on my well-being.

The place we stayed at provided guidance from coaches and shamans. The first two days, we engaged in extensive discussions about our intentions for the ceremony and what we could anticipate from it. We also did a lot of meditation and stretching along with a very strict diet.

Describing the events of the ceremony itself proves challenging, as the experience transcended ordinary expression. I heard the voices of my ancestors speaking to me in my mind, revealing that I had been carrying their accumulated trauma within my body. The leg pain, the discomfort in my head, and the intense morning anxiety all stemmed from their unresolved experiences. I questioned why this burden was necessary and requested permission to release it, as it no longer served a purpose in my life. Astonishingly, they granted me the ability to let it go. I simply needed to acknowledge its presence, express gratitude for the lessons it taught me, and ask for its release. Although it may sound peculiar, I can confidently say that since that transformative experience, I have not experienced any of those pains or anxiety again. This revelation occurred three months ago, and I continue to be free.

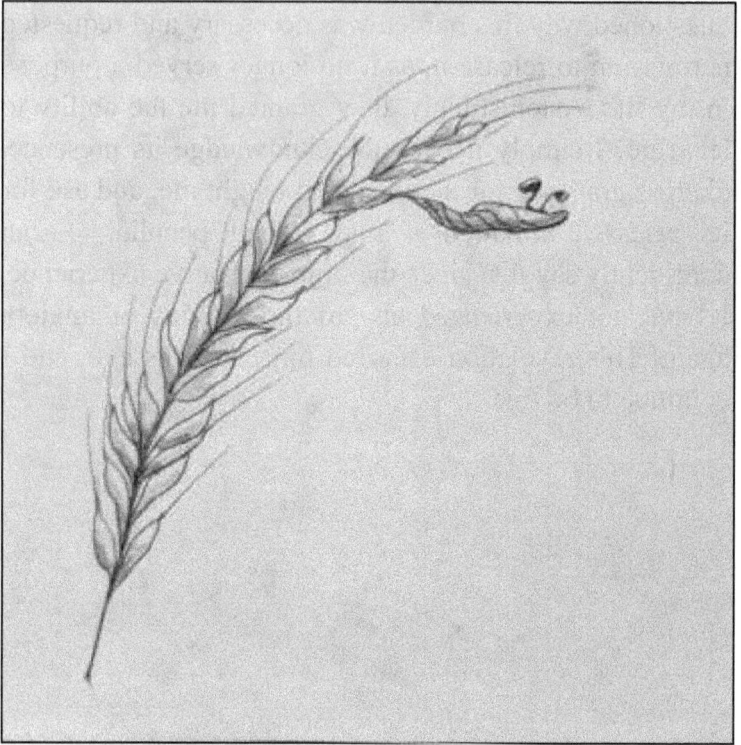

STORIES OF HEALING
EXPERIENCES WITH LAB-
BASED PSYCHEDELICS
LSD

LSD is a psychedelic compound derived from ergot; a fungus found in grains. It activates serotonin receptors in the brain, which produces changes in visual, auditory, and tactile perception. The psychedelic also promotes introspection and the dissolution of the "ego." LSD was first synthesized in 1938 by Swiss chemist Albert Hofmann, who accidentally discovered its psychedelic properties in 1947 when he accidentally ingested a small amount on what is now famously known as "Bicycle Day."

After learning that psychedelics induced hallucinations similar to those reported by schizophrenics, Dr. Humphry Osmond started researching the idea that mental illness could be caused by an imbalance of chemicals in the brain. Osmond was a psychiatrist at St. George's Hospital in London, and later practiced at the Saskatchewan Mental Hospital. His research on LSD led him to discover that a system of neurotransmitters with dedicated receptors might play a role in our mental experience. These findings ultimately contributed to the rise of neurochemistry in the 1950s and eventually led to the discovery of serotonin and the class of antidepressants known as SSRIs. [3] Contemporary research on LSD has revealed the psychedelic's potential to treat various psychiatric disorders. LSD has the ability to "reset" the default mode network, a series of brain processes that control our inner sense of self-worth and

[3] Dyck, Erika. *Psychedelic Psychiatry: LSD from Clinic to Campus.* Johns Hopkins University Press, 2008.

ego. Hyperactivity in the default mode network has been linked with depression, anxiety, obsessive compulsive disorder, addiction, and more. Stanislav Grof, a psychiatrist who was one of the pioneers of LSD assisted psychotherapy, predicted that psychedelics "would be for psychiatry what the microscope is for biology or the telescope is for astronomy." Grof found that under moderate doses of LSD his patients would connect better with the therapist, recover childhood traumas and give a voice to buried emotions.

In 2009, Robin Carhart-Harris, David Nutt, and Amanda Feilding were able to identify neural actions of a brain on psilocybin or LSD for the first time in history. Through the use of MRI's, Carhart-Harris observed that brain activity reduced in the default mode network while other areas of the brain lit up. This was compared to baseline imaging of the patient in a normal state. It is believed by many researchers that psychedelics can facilitate neuroplasticity. It is much easier for an individual to change a thought, brain pattern, or habit under the influence of psilocybin or LSD. Carhart-Harris's view is that even a temporary rewiring can bring lasting results, which is supported through scientific as well as anecdotal evidence.

Robert Jesse, a psychedelic researcher and advisor, recruited a group of experts in the mid-90s that eventually formed the psilocybin research team at Johns Hopkins. While doing research, Jesse found that there had been more than a thousand scientific papers on psychedelic drug therapy before 1965 with more than forty thousand research subjects. From the 1950's to early 1970's researchers were using psychedelic compounds to treat many conditions with impressive results.

In the mid-1950s, Bill Wilson–the cofounder of Alcoholics Anonymous (AA)–learned about Osmond and Hoffer's work with alcoholics. He went to Sidney Cohen, at the Brentwood VA hospital (and later UCLA) who had been researching LSD. There was a dozen or so groups in North America and Europe who were in close contact and sharing information. Wilson thought there was a place for LSD therapy in AA but his cohorts on the board disagreed, worried it would hurt the brand. Few members of AA realize that the whole idea of spiritual awakening leading one to surrender to a higher power–a cornerstone of AA– can be traced to psychedelics.

In 1965, CBS News had an hour-long report on LSD working for alcoholism titled *LSD: The Spring Grove Experiment*. The response was so positive that Maryland State established a multimillion-dollar research center at the Spring Grove State Hospital. Stan Graf, Walter Pahke and Bill Richards were hired to run it. It was shut down in the 1970's when their funds ran out and they lost government approval

LSD STORIES

Male / 43 / Amarillo / Sales

My problem was my temper, frustration level and having absolutely no patience. Anyone who knew me would tell you that. Don't get me wrong. I am a good guy and could temporarily hold it together when I was working, until I couldn't. One night my girlfriend of 16 years gave me a choice. So, I chose to go to someone she knew who did psychedelic therapy. Figured it was a fast fix from what people said. Turns out that was my impatience wanting everything yesterday-so fast fix was perfect. It is far from a fast fix BUT it is working. After 3 sessions in twelve weeks, I see remarkable changes in myself. My girlfriend is sticking around, so I assume she sees it too. Now, I am microdosing to continue a steady change. I have also calmed down enough to journal on a recording and talk with my guide once or twice a month. Before, my patience level wouldn't have allowed me to do either.

My job is going so much better and my sales are up. Writing up something like this would have never happened before. It would have taken too much of my time and patience. So yes ma'am, I would recommend this form of healing to everyone.

Female / 22 / Phoenix, AZ / Grad Student

Growing up in the foster care system had a lot of negative experiences. There were small and large traumas my whole life. Fortunately, my social worker and CASA volunteer were the best mentors for my future, hence being a Grad student at this point in my life. At the age of 21, my CASA volunteer confidentially told me about studies from the 1950s to 1970s that were being done on healing with LSD. She didn't recommend outright that I try it but she planted the seed. That set me down the road to read, read and read some more on the history of it.

Three months later I found someone who was doing work underground using LSD with their therapy. Lord knows how many regular therapists I have seen in my life but this was going to be different. I prayed. And it was. With the dose of LSD and a therapist in combination, it was shocking how much work was done in those four sessions. The LSD opened my subconscious without the trauma being activated in an overwhelming manner. So many circumstances came up and she coached me to 'stand my ground' in the situation while we talked through it. Her theory was to walk through the storm, resolve it with help and walk out the other side. It turned out to be an excellent protocol. We had sessions in between the LSD sessions to integrate what had occurred which was extremely helpful. Now I am feeling like I have a true handle on my own life. About 80% better which is a miracle. There isn't an ounce of hesitation to continue this work to become a better person. It has also helped me to change my path in life to become a therapist instead of my other focus of education. Hopefully I can help others like I was helped. Pass it on, if the whole world passed the generosity of others on what a wonderful world it would be!!

Female / 37 / Sonoma, CA / Preschool Teacher

I don't know why but I always felt something was wrong with me. I felt like my brain was so full of thoughts (mostly other people's opinions). Sometimes, I didn't feel like my brain was my own. I got the book at an airport that Michael Pollan wrote called How to Change Your Mind. It looked interesting and I had a long flight to S. Africa so I needed a book to keep me engaged. It was something that really wasn't on my radar but I am always trying to learn new things. By the time I finished it, I knew that I would try psychedelics when I returned to the U.S. (even though I knew they were a Schedule 1 drug).

The opportunity that I made happen by asking around was with LSD. There was a very well-known and respected woman in Berkeley who was willing to be my guide and therapist. Please know these brave souls are risking everything by doing this special work to help people. She could lose her license as a therapist and possibly spend time in jail. But she believes in the healing and helping of these substances. And they can help people like me and so she does it anyway. And she doesn't make a huge profit. It's not about the income. She spent all day with me for the price I normally pay for a couple of hours of regular therapy. The whole process was very intentional to make it as safe and as positive as possible.

My experience: During the trip it was like a road trip through my mind. I was the driver yet I moved to the passenger seat because I felt so trusting and safe. It was almost like a Disneyland ride going through different areas of my brain. I saw things from long ago that teachers, parents, adult neighbors, and other kids said to me. I felt how I felt at the time and noted how those things accumulated in my brain. It was an interesting feeling just driving around parts of my brain and memories. The emotions went from fear of the situations, the feeling that they knew better than me, to trying to please. Each time it took a little piece of my own self and replaced it with theirs. Eventually I came to the realization that I have a right to be my own self and honor what is me. I am valuable and deserve the space I take up in the world. If I speak my own truth, no one has the right to correct me or override it. What a liberating feeling!!

As the months have gone by and a few sessions with my psychedelic therapist, I have noticed that I no longer feel out of control in my own brain and thoughts. If there is something that comes up that doesn't sit well with me, I am able to easily work through it and know what my thought about it is. It sounds weird but I owe my sanity to LSD.

Male / 57 / Netherlands / Police Officer

With my job and the stress I was bringing home, I noticed I was drinking more and more. My wife kept telling me I was an alcoholic but of course I wouldn't admit to it. It started to affect my job so I had no choice but to find a resolution. Since I am an avid reader, I started reading everything I could about addictions. Living in the Netherlands where many drugs are legal, we are trained on them. But not so much on drinking abuse. There was a book about a man named Bill who started AA in America. It told how he found that LSD was 80%+ effective in 'curing' a drinking problem. Seemed like an easier thing for me to do (and quicker) than just trying to use my self-control. Being a police officer, it was easy (but maybe not legal the way I did it) to get some LSD. The thing that was a little harder was to find someone to guide me through the process. It took several weeks of quietly looking for a therapist who would help with the process and not document anything so it wouldn't be on my record.

Before the session, we spent a couple of weeks talking about my life and thoughts and what I was looking for. When the day came for the full day session, I was a bit nervous that it may not work and I was putting myself in this situation. Being an officer, we don't like to release control very easily.

The session was beautiful. The therapist guided me through it in a way not to steer anything but to help me relax into it. It lasted all day but I lost track of time completely. What I know is that after it was over, it seemed that drinking was unnecessary. I wondered why I ever even thought I needed a drink. There was so much more to life. Taking care of my health and body were so much more important. We had several talk sessions in the following weeks. It has been 18 months now. I still check in with the therapist about once a month but I have absolutely no craving at all. It has saved my career and most importantly, my marriage and family.

Female / 34 / Boston / Librarian

I had clinical depression for as long as I can remember. One day I was reading something about a trial using LSD to cure depression. I applied immediately. Willing to try anything at that point because NOTHING has worked for me. Besides multiple antidepressants, I never did a 'drug' in my life.

After several meetings of talk therapy and medical intakes, I had two full day sessions (one a week). Talk therapy in between and again after a few weeks. They set me up with a group to have weekly sessions. I keep a running diary, try to exercise more and have changed my diet. All because they recommended it and because after the LSD sessions, it was what I actually wanted to do.

It has been 9 months and my depression is so much gone that I no longer have that as a diagnosis on my medical chart. Life throws you curveballs but I can roll with it so much easier now and it doesn't send me down the well again. I am very grateful that I was accepted into that clinical trial. I am a completely different person because of it.

Male / 64 / Santa Fe, NM / Bakery Owner

LSD was familiar to me growing up but I never had personal experience with it. For the past few years, it seemed it was in a lot of conversations I was having. People were mentioning how it was helping them to feel like they belong to something greater than themselves. It seems that the world is becoming a lonelier place with all the technology and people are craving personal connections. It really is a basic human need that we were biologically designed for. It wasn't possible to survive thousands of years ago on our own. As a businessman, I am speaking with people all day, every day. But it's not what you would call my community. It's just the way I have to make my living. To me, it's almost worse being around people all the time yet feeling disconnected.

It was pretty easy to find an intentional group that was using LSD for a tool to connect with the universe and each other. It was also easy for me to make the decision to join them in a ceremony. What my story is about is how so very much I gained from doing that ceremony. It has given me a community of people who want to be connected and support each other. The feeling I got from my three ceremonies was what I can only explain as a universal mind, a one consciousness. That we are all connected rather we know it or feel it. It was the most loving, connectedness that words can't even begin to explain. I am no longer lonely-EVER. Everyone should do this. There wouldn't be any more hate, war or crime because people would realize they are only doing it to themselves.

Male / 34 / Orlando, FL / Delivery Driver

"Everyone was doing it", so I heard. With my need to be in the know, I also had to try it. I didn't really think that I needed it but everyone says they get something from it. So, my intention wasn't really to heal but that's exactly what my experience gave me in an odd way.

It was easy to get since everyone is doing it. I read a lot about it and found someone to sit with me just to be safe. Just in case I was one of those that we all learned about in the anti-drug education programs in school who jumped off a roof or went crazy. I also took the advice of "go slow, start low".

I wouldn't say I was a shallow person but after doing LSD, I realized I was just very unaware. My sitter had a music playlist and I also decided to "go inside" for this experience. I wore an eye mask so I would be in my own world, not part of what was going on around me. This was my experience: I NEVER noticed the beauty of music before. I didn't know the songs, yet they REALLY touched me emotionally. I felt a part of the music which also gave me the feeling of being a part of something so much bigger on a universal level. The whole experience seemed like I WAS the music playing in the whole cosmos. Which all just sounds so trippy when written down. It's one of those experiences that you just had to be there. What is a very important note (sorry, not supposed to be a pun) is that the aftereffects were how much more aware and grateful I became for beauty. I notice trees, flowers, music, the sky and people's emotions in their faces in detail. Before I never REALLY looked at things.

This is a huge gift to me and I am sure to others that I am around because I SEE them now. My opinion-everyone should do it once (safely of course).

Female / 50 / New York / Interior Designer

The first time I tried LSD, I was young. It was with a group of safe friends. We felt such a part of everything and everything was beautiful. There was such a connection we had with each other. The next time was at a Grateful Dead concert with too much stimulation. We got separated and I ended up in a situation that immediately filled me with high anxiety and fear. That was a wake-up call. Now I realize that it is very important to be very intentional because these are powerful healing products that can really help or do damage. This is my message to spread. Take them seriously and there can be a beautiful experience. Take them in the wrong setting and it can be traumatic and you can find yourself in a bad situation. Respect them and they will respect you.

Male / 62 / New York, NY / Stock Market Analyst

After working with a therapist who used Internal Family Systems for about 6 months. We got on the subject of how psychedelics were being used in combination with IFS therapy. She said the findings were very favorable. She didn't work with psychedelics but had a colleague that did. What the plan was to have all three of us together. Each one of them would be doing the part that was their expertise. I was not sure about how successful the outcome would be for me but trusted my therapist.

It was an all-day 'treatment'. I took the LSD after quite a bit of intention setting and some stretching. We all decided it was best to start slow with a 'more isn't better' attitude. That made me a lot more comfortable. Plus, I didn't want to be overwhelmed with whatever was going to come my way. After a while (no idea how long or of time during the day) my body and brain started to loosen up. Thoughts that had never occurred to me arose. When I talked through what was happening, my therapist was able to use the IFS therapy to really help these thoughts and voices. It was like I was attending a huge family reunion of people I didn't know existed but they all lived in me. Everyone wanted to tell their story. I needed to hear and figure out all those stories coming through. Without my therapist, when I was thinking about it afterwards, it would have been just utter chaos. There might have been some revelations coming from it but with her help I feel it was an almost overwhelming amount of healing in one day. Not complaining -just amazed! There were so many parts of me that had been locked in a dungeon no wonder I didn't even know who I was. Usually, I was the person who I was with. Just a chameleon. Which is why I went to therapy in the first place. At 62, I was wondering who I really was.

This type of combination was an enormous help to me. We have plans to possibly do it again in six months if I feel everything has been worked through from that healing day. And if we feel I even need that kind of help again. Now, I can tell you who I (me, myself) is, what I want and am starting to have awareness when it isn't me or MY thought/wish/problem. It's so great to get to know ME.

Male / 73 / Pensacola, FL / Retired CEO

At the golf club of all places, there was a conversation about a man and his wife doing an MDMA session together. Isn't that a nightclub drug?! He explained it was different and this session was used for the intention of healing a marriage relationship of 40 years. It was a very interesting and enlightening conversation. I went home and read everything I could find about it. My marriage of 38 years was just a contract but probably most of the fault of my own. All the years of travel and not being home much. My family and wife were virtually ignored my whole career. I wanted more of my marriage and life at this golden stage of my life.

What my studies taught me is that MDMA is an amphetamine and can-do things to the heart. At 73, I wasn't willing to risk a heart attack. What I did find out is that LSD works more through the brain and not the body so that was my final choice. The acquaintance at the golf club was able to connect me with someone who worked with LSD and she was a psychiatrist working underground. Lord, bless these people who risk everything to help heal the world!

After three LSD sessions plus sober sessions my wife was so impressed by the changes in me that she started going! It has been a life changer for us and our marriage. It is like we are newly married honeymooners. We remembered why we chose each other. Our kids are stunned and can't understand what happened to us. Of course, we haven't told them the details other than we were seeing a psychiatrist. Maybe someday when they are married or have marital problems, we will share with them.

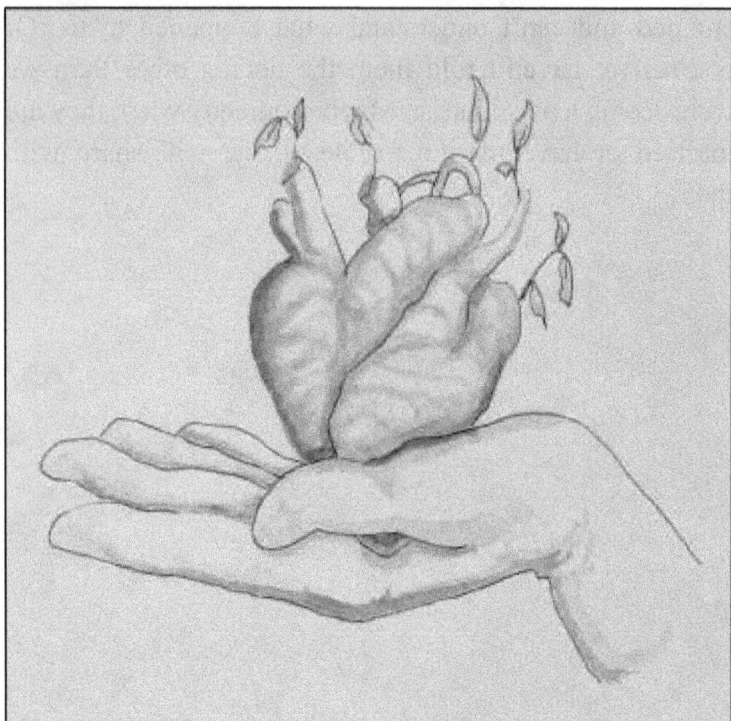

STORIES OF HEALING EXPERIENCES WITH LAB-BASED PSYCHEDELICS
MDMA

MDMA (3,4-Methylenedioxymethamphetamine) is a synthetic drug in the amphetamine class of compounds. This synthetic, psychoactive substance is best known for producing a euphoric state with simultaneous stimulant and psychedelic effects. Its effects are produced by increasing the levels of serotonin, dopamine and norepinephrine in the brain.

MDMA was first synthesized in 1912 by a Merck chemist, Anton Köllisch. At the time, Merck was interested in developing substances that stopped abnormal bleeding. Originally called "Methylsafrylaminc," the scientists were unable to find a practical use for it. Nevertheless, in 1914, they patented the substance as something that could one day have therapeutic value, and then shelved it, leaving MDMA to be forgotten for decades. Then in the 1950s and 1960s, it was tested by the United States as a potential mind-control drug or truth serum.

The most famous series of experiments was the CIA's Project MK-Ultra. Though most documents from that time period were destroyed following a death in the program, some survive today. According to these official documents, MDMA was never tested in humans, only animals. A compound called MDE, which is almost identical to MDMA, was tested on humans at the New York State Psychiatric Institute.[4] In the 1970s, MDMA

---

[4] Hallifax, James. "A Brief History of MDMA: From the

became a popular adjunct to psychotherapy due to its empathogenic qualities that help patients open up and form a bond with their therapists. Empathogens refers to a category of drugs that produce heightened senses of empathy and compassion toward others and self.

It is important to note that pure MDMA is not the same as Molly or Ecstasy, which are considered "club drugs" and may contain highly toxic additives. Unlike Molly or Ecstasy, pure MDMA has been considered an important therapeutic drug for the treatment of PTSD, anxiety, depression, and other mental health disorders since the 1970s and 80s. MDMA was made illegal in 1985, however, after the substance leaked from the clinic and started circulating around in the mainstream public.

Despite the criminalization of MDMA, according to the 2021 National Survey on Drug Use and Health, roughly 2.2 million people reported using MDMA at least once over the past 12 months. Dr. Gul Dolen, neuroscientist and professor at Johns Hopkins–and the chief investigator at Dolen LAB in Baltimore–provided conclusive evidence that MDMA could reopen critical learning periods, effectively reverting the adult brain back into an adolescent brain through reorganizing the extracellular matrix and the network of synaptic plasticity for a few hours to a couple of weeks. Dr. Dolen has also conducted some interesting research on

---

CIA to Raves to Psychedelic Therapy." *Psychedelic Spotlight*, 2 June 2024. psychedelicspotlight.com/history-of-mdma-cia-ravespsychedelic-therapy/

MDMA and octopi. Normally an octopus is very territorial and a solitary creature, but when given MDMA, this was not the case. Today, approved clinics are using MDMA in the treatment of PTSD, depression, anxiety, autism spectrum disorder, and other mental health disorders. MDMA is also being utilized in couples therapy as well for its ability to break down biases and promote a sense of empathy and connection between partners. MAPS, the Multidisciplinary Association for Psychedelic Studies, is a not-for-profit research development company that is sponsoring a lot of these trials worldwide. These trials mainly consist of preparatory sessions followed by a 6–8-hour treatment session with MDMA. The patients also participate in follow-up sessions to emotionally, mentally, and spiritually process their experience, and to repeat it as necessary.

MDMA STORIES

Male / 58 / Consultant / USA

I grew up in a family of 4 boys, all engineers. We were a very cognitive group and our family structure rewarded thinking over feeling. In fact, in hindsight, my parents for their own reason weren't well equipped for holding and honoring emotions or helping us navigate them.

My first opening happened with MDMA. This heart opening experience transformed me and confirmed what I knew internally but what wasn't always supported in my family. How to engage life from my heart vs. my head.

These experiences were the cracking in my mind/heart that offered a beautiful new way to perceive my life, feel myself and connect to others. I got to observe, in a very non-judgmental way, the patterns of my life and how they constricted me. This very deep inner experience showed me, in a short order, where change was needed in my life and with support of a guide, how I could start to change.

There have been many journeys since my first. I now realize this process for me is not a one-time event but instead is a lifelong journey of opening, change, learning and humility to what life is and has to offer. And I'm good with this and I'm happy to know life will never be boring. The journey continues

Female / 32 / Melbourne, Australia / Supervisor

My interest in MDMA was for the purpose of shifting burnout from life's stresses, childhood PTSD, OCD and panic attacks. I had read it could help all of those. It is now legal in Australia with a therapist but it was over $10,000 for each session. My only other way to turn was underground, which seems crazy because it is legal now - albeit extremely unaffordable. It was easy to find someone who had a lot of really good references. Which I should point out is VERY important. We both had a connection upon meeting. We had a few talk sessions and then it was MDMA day.

My words will not be able to truly articulate what I want to say so please forgive me. I can't give you a 'trip report' because it would sound too crazy. But it wasn't scary (after the trip started, before I was extremely nervous). What doesn't sound crazy is that the aftermath of what I was shown/told/felt is that all of my psychosis was dialed down about 5 notches. I just seemed to have this sense of calmness and peace that really helped EVERYTHING.

When it came time 3 months later to do it again, I was still nervous even though I kind of knew what to expect. Another 5 notches of relief occurred. It has now been one year and 4 sessions later. I can't begin to understand how I even lived in my brain the way I was. Survival I suppose and I didn't know anything else except that I didn't like having all those issues. Bless the people who have the courage to practice this underground because so many people like myself can benefit. It wasn't all the MDMA, don't get me wrong. I had a LOT of work to do but it was such a brilliant tool in helping me. And, I still haven't come near paying $10,000 for all the sessions I have had. Although healing is priceless, it's just a matter of being able to afford it. True healers are not in it to get rich. This is about healing and helping humanity.

Married Couple / 51 & 54 / Business Owners

After being married for 30 years we had just become more like roommates. We own a business and also work together which takes a lot of romance out of a relationship. Some close friends of ours shared one night at dinner that they did some marriage counseling in combination with MDMA. Honestly, we were shocked. They were the most prim and proper couple we knew. What were they doing taking dance club drugs?!? Since we were basically speechless, we just listened. They shared with us that it was like they were honeymooners again. That MDMA in its pure form is not like street drugs. Taking that combined talking with a marriage counselor they were able to talk freely, that it literally closed down their egos. They were both able to share what was on their minds for quite some time. Hurts, not feeling heard or respected and a list of other things. They said it bonded them in a way they never imagined and ignited their dud sex life.

This is supposed to be our story we are sharing so here we go. We got the name of the counselor and made an appointment. If they were recommending it, we thought that was good enough for us. We had a couple of sessions so we could all get to know each other and she would know about our history and issues. The day came and it was the most beautiful day of our lives. The love in the room, the care, concern, and non-judgmental conversations were amazing. We walked out of there like it was our wedding day. And my husband is not embarrassed to tell you, our wedding night. We have never been that hot for each other even when it was a new relationship. Not sure why the sexual physical part turned on but we both love it. And we are extremely happy we took this adventure together. Absolutely we would do it again if we ever felt it was necessary. We still see our counselor occasionally as she is helping our new habits of communication stick so we don't get lazy and go back to how it was.

Male / 31 / Alaska / Float Plane Pilot

After reading about a study done by Professor Gul Dolen with octopus and MDMA, I was addicted to learning about this new (to me) drug. What the research found was when octopuses were given MDMA, they became uncharacteristically social and playful. Which is what I have craved for my own life. I suffer from extreme shyness but feel like there is play in me that really wants to come out. I started asking around if anyone knew how I could be part of a study or find an underground therapist to try taking MDMA. It took a while but the opportunity finally came to try it in a safe situation with a trained therapist (albeit illegally underground). Four sessions and 2 years later (the first being the most incredible) I am quite a different person. Still on the quiet side but much more social and I am not so 'held back' to let myself have fun and be playful.

Female / 60 / Seattle / Chef

I grew up with what people called childhood neglect. Of course, you don't realize it as a child but you grow up knowing or feeling you are broken somehow. My life just kept getting worse and worse no matter what type of traditional healing I tried. It got to the point psychedelics were my last hope.

My guide was an angel. I was very scared but knew it needed to happen. The MDMA was so good to me. Never in my life had I ever been still. I was always doing, proving, earning my keep…For the entire day, I just laid on her couch loving myself. The message that kept coming over and over is, "just be". That was such a radical thought for me…".JUST BE. I am a child of God, I am loved, I am valuable. I don't need to 'do' to show my worth".

That was 2 years ago and the feeling hasn't left me yet. Sometimes I get a little too busy but am immediately aware and ask myself the intention for the "busy". No longer does the feeling of having to earn my value, love or proving myself dominate my life. I am still working on myself but that was such a huge help up. It all doesn't seem so overwhelming now.

Male / 75 / USA / Retired Mail Carrier

This is a story about my uncle. He suffered a series of strokes and, unfortunately, wasn't able to receive effective medical treatment until the critical recovery window had passed. Desperate to find something that could help him recover, I sought advice from countless doctors and medical providers. Eventually, someone suggested that I apply for a new clinical trial using MDMA to treat stroke victims.

The application process took a couple of months, and every day that passed felt excruciating, knowing that time is crucial in stroke recovery. It was a tremendous relief when he was finally accepted into the study. The trial specifically targeted individuals who were well past the traditional recovery period, offering hope where little had been left.

What happened next was nothing short of extraordinary. He regained a remarkable amount of function. The explanation given was that MDMA helps restore brain plasticity. Essentially temporarily turning back the clock to a time of youthful brain health. During the treatment, he worked with a physical therapist, and somehow, the combination enabled his brain to start functioning properly again. There are detailed scientific explanations for why it worked, rooted in neurology, which I appreciate but don't entirely understand.

What I do know is that I am profoundly grateful. My uncle now has a quality of life again and is almost back to his old self.

Female / 72 / Iowa / Retired Social Worker

I was soooo nervous but felt this was my last hope. Right before I took the "heart medicine" my question to my coach was, "is this addicting?" She assured me it was not. Even though every advertisement and story about MDMA was that it caused immediate addiction and it turned your brain into Swiss cheese. I was willing anyway, because of my desperation for my life to continue.

After the day of the most beautiful experience of my life, it ended. The feeling in my entire being was LOVE. BUT I had no intention of doing it anytime soon or again. So, NO not addicting. And if the Swiss cheese brain feels like abundant love, then, I LOVE Swiss cheese.

It is amazing how severe depression is tied to lack of feeling and giving love. This was like God coming down and kissing me on the top of the head. That was 10 weeks ago and I am still buzzing with emotions I have never felt. The protocol is 3 times but some people wait many months in between. I don't know when the calling to do it again will come. Whenever that is, I will answer the call!

Husband & Wife / 43 & 52 / Croatia Professionals

We were having bad marriage problems. We loved each other but just couldn't get our relationship together. During our therapy sessions we would end up shouting at each other the whole time. One day, I was reading about therapy for couples that were assisted with MDMA and the therapist. Since we were most likely ending our relationship, it was worth a try. Finding someone was difficult. Especially a 'qualified' person to lead us.

MDMA opened our hearts. Our conversations were love filled and no offense was taken when the other person said their side. It was like someone put our egos in a box and only let love in the conversation. The amount of listening and being heard was so incredible. This has helped our marriage to go from a 1-star to a 4-star (out of 5) in just one appointment. Now we can go to therapy and actually accomplish something. Maybe another one of these appointments will be in our future but for now, it gave us an enormous jumpstart!!!

Female / 32 / East Coast, US / Army Medic

After being in the military and seeing some pretty gruesome shit my drinking habits really escalated. A few drinks at the end of the day, when possible, to every night about 12 drinks when I got back stateside. I knew it wasn't healthy and I couldn't stop. A friend of mine heard about a study for military personnel who had served. It was a 2-month commitment with therapy sessions and 2 MDMA sessions. The study was taking MDMA under therapeutic conditions to reduce alcohol consumption/misuse. Lucky for me, I was accepted into the study. The talking sessions brought out a lot of PTSD that I didn't even realize I had. The MDMA sessions brought so much clarity, self-love and forgiveness. It was interesting how when on the MDMA I was able to relive some things that had caused me huge amounts of anxiety. But it seemed I was an observer and able to just watch and think about those situations rationally. They told me it was actually rewiring my brain. The PTSD made my brain use the amygdala and the thinking part was cut off.

After the study I feel so much calmer and aware. I didn't realize that I hadn't been aware of much at all. Most of my thinking was around just surviving. I will still have a very occasional drink with friends but it is not a problem anymore. The awareness lets me know when to stop or not even start - and usually after just one beer.

Male / 29 / Colorado / Mechanic

Interesting fact I read in an article is that all tears are not the same. Tears cried with joy have a different chemical structure than sad tears or onion tears. Scientists can look at the tears without the person near and tell you what they are about. Which is so crazy to me because sometimes we aren't even sure what the tears are about when they are coming out of our own eyes. At least I didn't.

All of my life, I have been THAT person that cried too easily. Commercials, movies, a cute puppy on the street, being turned down by a female…. It was quite embarrassing even though I did get pretty good at covering it up. The odd thing is that I would not consider myself an emotional person. Most of the time, I couldn't tell you if I was mad, sad or frustrated. A friend gave me a Brene Brown book on emotions. It was very helpful having a go-to book to try to find what I was feeling. I actually made flashcards from its descriptions. Wow, this all really makes me look like a dufus. But by telling all this, it shows me and the reader how much I needed some heart healing. This same friend was doing an MDMA study for depression. She told me that it works for all kinds of issues that they are studying. So, I started reading everything I could about it. It turns out that MDMA is known as the "heart medicine" because it helps to open the heart up.

It wasn't hard to find an underground coach who was using MDMA to help people. He came with a lot of great recommendations which were very important to me. And he wasn't trying to make his fortune. He was very affordable for me. At our first meeting we had a great connection and I felt secure with him and the MDMA he was using. He said it was always tried first by the leaders in his community before they shared it with clients. After two talk sessions beforehand, we set a date. He encouraged me to clear my schedule for at least a day or two after so I could process and integrate with his help. Jumping right back into traffic and work can erase a lot of the work. Since I was taking time to do this, I wanted it to be as successful as possible.

The day was so much more than I could have wished for. It felt like there was layer after layer of armor, brick and mortar just melting away. I cried all day. Tears of release and relief. Who knew how much we can build up around the heart so we can't even access it even if we tried and wanted to. When it was almost over, I felt the most beautiful emerald light just pouring into my heart area, filling it up. Filling it up with healing and beauty where there was solid concrete before.

I still cry easily but now I can identify why and mostly it's from joy and gratitude. No question if I would do it again. It was the most spiritual, love filled day of my life. I don't feel like I HAVE to do it again but when it's time, I won't hesitate.

Female / 47 / USA / Teacher

My aunt was in her last days of life. The family was struggling because she was much too young to die of the big C. She was so scared of death. The doctor told us of a study for end-of-life cancer patients. It was taking a drug called MDMA. My aunt never took a drug in her life but she was so much more fearful of death than this so-called party drug. We were educated on how MDMA in a pure form is nothing like the party drugs kids take. It was amazing and surprising that they let us stay in the room while the therapist gave her the MDMA. After about 40 minutes she really perked up. She had been really groggy and not really there from the pain medications she was on for the last couple of weeks. It was such a gift that she was able to really communicate with us. She had never been an emotional or open person but told us how much she deeply loved us. She opened up about a lot with the family that was there. It actually turned her death into a beautiful, peaceful, loving event. Her last comment was that she wasn't afraid to die and leave. She saw there was something more and she was actually looking forward to it. So, the MDMA not only helped her on her last days, it helped all of us. We all have a very different view of death now.

Female /52 / East Coast USA / Permaculturist

For more years than I care to think about, I have struggled. My childhood didn't seem 'that bad' until I started telling stories out loud to my many many therapists. Then it seemed horrible. No wonder I was such a mess. Depression, anxiety, several mysterious illnesses that no one could ever figure out…You name it, I tried it. From natural herbs to psychics to specialists in mainstream medicine. Money, time, frustration, loss of hope was very quickly gaining on me.

One night in one of my support groups, a woman took me aside and suggested I try MDMA. She knew a psychedelic therapist who could help me safely. It was so out of my realm but my first instinct was, "what the hell do I have to lose". I am not naïve so before I called her, I did some research so I would have an idea of what to expect. Ha! I didn't expect AT ALL what happened. BUT, it was the most beautiful experience of my life. It did for me what 30 years of all the other things combined couldn't do. Somehow, it 'released me'. It showed me I don't need all the walls, worry, control or proving. Believe me, I am still doing the work but it is like I have lost 100 pounds of sickness. That was 9 months ago and I can still access the feelings of that day. I journal, meditate, talk to my psychedelic coach occasionally and joined a psychedelic support group. It's not a magic potion BUT it sure gives you a huge hand up out of the muck. I may do another session again but feel like so far, I don't need it, it still hasn't 'left' me.

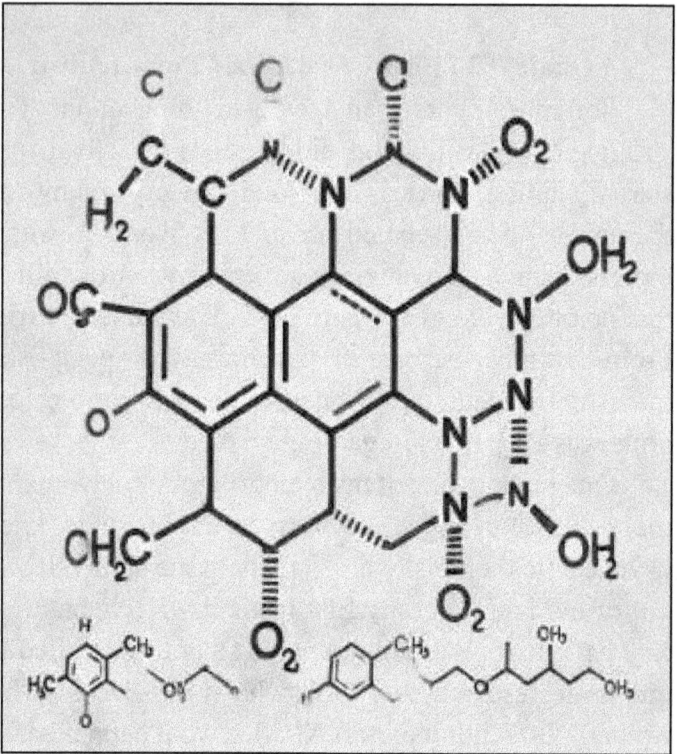

STORIES OF HEALING
EXPERIENCES WITH LAB-
BASED PSYCHEDELICS
Ketamine

Ketamine is classified as a dissociative hallucinogenic, meaning it distorts the perception of sights and sounds, as well as emotions and personal identification of self. It doesn't directly block pain signals like an opiate. Instead, dissociative analgesics disconnect the thalamus from the cortex. When this happens, the body still feels pain, but the brain doesn't register it. Unlike most drugs, ketamine targets many different receptors at once, making it very difficult to understand exactly what's going on or how it works.[5]

Chronic stress depletes the synapses in certain regions of the brain, — especially the medial prefrontal cortex. This region is often implicated in the effects of depression which bolster the effects of BDNF and mTORC1, which are ultimately responsible for the regrowth of synapses.[6]

Ketamine was approved by the FDA in 1970 as a surgical anesthetic and analgesic, and has been listed on the World Health Organization's List of Essential Medicines since 1985. When used ketamine is given

---

[5] Visser, E. and S.A. Schug. "The Role of Ketamine in Pain Management." *Biomedicine & Pharmacotherapy = Biomedecine & Pharmacotherapie* vol. 60,7 (2006): 341-8. doi:10.1016/j.biopha.2006.06.021

[6] Li, Linda, and Phillip E. Vlisides. "Ketamine: 50 Years of Modulating the Mind." *Frontiers in Human Neuroscience* vol. 10 612. 29 Nov. 2016, doi:10.3389/fnhum.2016.00612

as an intravenous injection (IV), as an intramuscular injection, lozenge, or a nasal spray. Studies have shown that ketamine regulates blood sugar levels in regions of the brain associated with depression, while also stimulating the growth of synapses. It opens a window of neuroplasticity, so what you do before, during, and after each session impacts your experience and results. Ketamine therapy, or ketamine-assisted therapy, is a mental health treatment that uses low doses of ketamine for treatment-resistant depression, anxiety disorders, substance abuse disorders and PTSD (posttraumatic stress disorder).

It is believed to allow neurons to form new connections and fire together in ways that create novel pathways in the brain (called brain plasticity or neuroplasticity). In depression, the brain's ability to make connections is impaired. Ketamine reboots this ability and wakes up the dormant, depressed brain. In addition, ketamine therapy may also help turn off a stressed-out state that the brain can get stuck in.[7]

During psychotherapy sessions with ketamine, patients are on ketamine while talking with a therapist. These are generally 2-to-3-hour sessions. A

---

[7] Migala, Jessica. "What Is Ketamine Therapy? Risks, Benefits, Effectiveness, and More." *EverydayHealth.Com*, 18 Aug. 2023, www.everydayhealth.com/integrative-health/ketamine-therapy/guide/.

prescription ketamine spray called Spravato® is also currently on the market for treatment-resistant depression, or depression that doesn't improve with conventional medications. Some insurances cover Spravato and sessions like preparation and integration as well as the medicine sessions. Many providers use traditional ketamine off label, which is usually not covered by insurance. Sometimes preparation and integration sessions are covered by insurance companies even when ketamine off label is used, it totally depends on the insurance company. There are also stipulations about how many sessions a person can have. It is a messy and confusing system. Although there is an abundance of scientific evidence to support the benefits of ketamine, there's still resistance to this substance as it is associated with abuse. With more clinical research, scientists hope to better understand ketamine and its ability to help people with mental health diagnoses.[8]

---

[8] Hasty, Marie. "Who Can Benefit from Ketamine Therapy? Psychedelic Support." *Psychedelic Support,* 19 Aug. 2024, psychedelic.support/resources/who-can-benefit-from-ketamine-therapy/.

KETAMINE STORIES

Female / 41 / East Coast USA / Sales Rep

I had absolutely no emotions ever since I can remember. Shut down. No ups or downs. When people cried at weddings, funerals or movies I just didn't get it. Why was I this way? I don't know but I felt like something must be terribly wrong with me. Especially when I got in a relationship and was told by my partner that very same thing. He suggested I try Ketamine assisted therapy. He raved how it worked for him and his problems. Mostly to keep our relationship, I made an appointment. The first time I went, nothing happened to speak of. The second time, I didn't remember much of it. But the third, fourth and fifth times, I sobbed and sobbed and sobbed. It felt so good. Not sure what it was all about but it opened something in me. Now, I cry very easily. Almost embarrassingly easily. But for now, I will take it. Because with the tears came the joy. The tears seemed to release, clean something out and make room for joy and feelings of happiness. I will be damned if I can explain it with words but that's ok because I spent my life using words in place of feeling.

Female / 28 / Phoenix, AZ / Tattoo Artist

My story is about a struggle with postpartum depression after the birth of my first child. It was a very traumatic birth to say the least. Lots of mistakes by the hospital staff and my doctor. The depression started the minute I walked back into our house with this beautiful new soul. When I called my doctor a week later, I was dismissed with the words that I had a healthy baby-everything turned out fine in the end, I should be grateful for that. Everyone else I opened up to basically said the same.

No one around was willing to listen to my 'whining' because my baby in my arms showed everything was alright. On the outside maybe, but I needed to process what had happened. I wasn't prepared at all even though I took all the classes and read all the books. Luckily, I came upon an article that Kate Kincade out of Tucson AZ wrote. She is a researcher with psychedelic healing. What she wrote stunned me. It was everything I just mentioned above. Her clinic is using Ketamine to help with Postpartum depression. A REAL stigma for a nursing mother!!

I wanted to be around for this baby and be the best mother I could. I contacted her clinic and had a great discussion with them. So, to cut to the chase, I went to Tucson several times and did a series of therapist-led 2.5-hour sessions with Ketamine. It meant I couldn't feed my baby for a minimum of 12 hours after, but I pumped to discard the milk so I could continue what I had my heart set on which was to nurse my baby.

OH MY GOD - THANK YOU!!! It was just what I needed. To release that trauma and the postpartum de pression with help by a caring listening professional. Worth every penny!!

Male / 33 / Berkeley, CA / Business Owner

Therapy didn't work for me. I was too shut down— or maybe I just didn't know where to begin. SSRIs didn't help either. One day I came across an article from a well-known research hospital discussing how Ketamine combined with talk therapy was showing highly positive results. Intrigued, I sought out a clinic following this protocol.

The sessions are long, sometimes lasting up to three hours, but they've been incredibly effective. It's remarkable how my brain opens up during the process, almost instinctively identifying what I need to work on with my therapist. She's skilled at guiding me, helping me unlock feelings, memories, and deeper insights. Without the usual resistance, the progress feels profound.

I've completed three sessions so far, and they've accomplished more for me than years of traditional approaches. I feel lighter, happier, and more connected to my emotions, which now seem so much easier to access. This is a path of healing I plan to continue, and yes, I wholeheartedly recommend it to others seeking deeper emotional breakthroughs.

Male / 44 / Concord, CA / Software Designer

I spent about eight years in traditional therapy, but it always felt like I was just going in circles, rehashing my history. It wasn't working, but I didn't know what else to try. Then I came across a report about combining therapy with Ketamine. Intrigued, I started researching and found a treatment center I could access. After speaking with them and learning about their protocol, I decided to give it a shot.

Their approach included an initial talk therapy session, followed by six sessions integrating Ketamine. After just the first two combination sessions, I was blown away by how much more effective it was! The Ketamine seemed to break the cycle of repetitive conversations that had defined the past eight years of therapy. It "unstuck" my brain, allowing me to dig deeper. When my therapist asked questions, I found myself offering new, more meaningful answers—answers that felt truly helpful.

By the time I completed five sessions, I realized I had accomplished more than in nearly a decade of traditional therapy. The process has been transformative. For years, I felt like a part of me was missing, but I couldn't figure out what it was. It felt like my brain was stuck behind a locked gate, unable to access what I needed. Ketamine opened that gate, giving me access to my thoughts, awareness, and the questions I should have been exploring all along.

I have one more session to go, and my hope is that it will bring a sense of completion. I'm so grateful I found this treatment—it has been nothing short of amazing.

Female / 68 / Las Vegas / Retired Designer

Struggling with depression for a large part of my life gave me the opportunity to try every drug out there that they could prescribe me. Therapy sessions for decades didn't seem to accomplish anything but repeatedly going over and over 'my problems'. I guess I am one of those people that don't need/want to discuss things over and over and over. To me, it seemed that was what kept me stuck in 'that' place.

One of my friends started ketamine treatments and it was like someone switched her back on. So off I went to try to get the same magic. It's very expensive and they recommend that you need 6 sessions to start. But I was thinking of how much money I spent on furniture, clothes, good wine….and this was going to help me hopefully. Hopefulness is a good thing. It's what gave me the little shove I needed to invest in myself.

It turned out to be the best investment I have ever made. The sessions along with the therapy really cracked something open that was in a vault inside me. Everything is easier. Even the hard things. I heard someone once say, "a smooth brain". That's how my brain feels now. All the jagged sharp edges have been filed down. I can't really explain in doctor terms how it works but for me it did. I wouldn't hesitate to do more sessions to continue my new smooth brain experience.

Male / 72 / Eugene, OR / Retired Fire Chief

You can only imagine the things I've seen in my career, things that would haunt your worst nightmares. Those images seemed to stick and pile up as I got older. My career as a first responder was very fulfilling, but eventually, it took a toll on my mental health. Fortunately, I was close to retirement and decided to leave a little early. I had access to excellent mental healthcare and genuinely tried to get better. However, all the talking seemed to ignite the PTSD that had accumulated over the years.

Finally, a doctor recommended ketamine treatments. Following his suggestion, I went to try it. After the first session, I walked out thinking, "What the hell was that?!" But after discussing it with a therapist, he encouraged me to continue. I'm glad I did. It took a few sessions to get used to it and relax, but that's when the progress started. When I stopped fighting and trying to control everything, the treatment was able to show me what I needed. And the therapist who was very familiar with Ketamine was a huge part of helping me.

For someone who had never done any drugs and didn't know anyone who did, this was a huge leap of faith. My advice to my younger self would be to let go and allow someone or something else to take charge. Be a receiver, not always the rescuer. My diagnosis is no longer PTSD, and I will continue on this path as appropriate.

Female / 29 / Ontario / Stay-at-home mom

My story is that I was drinking far too much to be taking good care of my children. I tried to stop but didn't have the willpower. One day I was reading about a study that was going to take place with Ketamine regarding alcoholism. It had psychological therapy attached to it also. I am so thankful I was accepted for that program. What happened was that I had to go to several sessions of therapy first. Then the next 3 times that I went, I got Ketamine in an IV and therapy at the same time. It was the best therapy session I have ever experienced. It kind of made me feel a bit detached from my story so when I told it, I didn't have the normal feelings attached to it. It made it so easy for my mind to look at the story in another light. The therapist was wonderful. He was able to get me to dive deeper than I could have imagined. My story no longer seemed relevant to my life now. After it was over, I just felt like I was so much more everything than I had ever given myself credit for. I continued therapy for several more appointments after the study. My drinking problem has completely changed. I can have a glass of wine once in a while but no longer crave it. If I never had a drink again, I think I would be happy. But I am glad that I can drink occasionally and not go overboard. AA should be using this!!

Female / 32 /Austin, TX / Musician

I had a lot of aches and pains for a 32-year-old. A lot of female issues. So much so, it made me dislike being a woman. My therapist suggested Ketamine. She said it might help me 'sort some things out'. I really wasn't even sure what there was to sort out or how to begin. Talk therapy went on for years but nothing changed. So why not try this new thing. What it ended up doing for me (so I can make my very long story short). The bottom line is it helped me heal the relationship I had with my body. I was my own worst enemy. Hating my body because of the aches and pains and 'sickness' it brought. This magic K medicine (with a LOT of my help- doing all the things they tell you to do) has helped me be a kind, gentle friend to myself instead. And my body is thanking me for that. It just needed to feel loved and not the enemy I was always fighting with. Getting rid of a lot of things I was holding onto in my brain and heart most likely also had a lot to do with it. Since then, I have read a book called, *The Body Keeps Score*. It explains how we hold onto all the crap and that can make our bodies sick.

Male / 38 / Houston, TX / Financial Planner

Friend or foe? This discussion has been coming up lately in my psychedelic men's circle. I definitely say friend. Ketamine has changed my life (sounds so cliché). Some said foe because they were concerned it was a crutch. Well, when you break a leg, what is wrong with using a crutch until you heal?!? Same thing, is my argument. If my leg healed and I insisted on taking the crutch with me every day for years, maybe that would be a foe. But until then, I am thankful I can use this medicine for healing old wounds, which is helping my temper and frustration. But most importantly becoming a better man for my family.

Female / 62 / CA / Mother

Yesterday in my journey I sat at the exact exquisite pinpoint of all that is possible to experience in this human life. I sat at the juncture of pain and love, and I sat there for the longest time. Waves of grief and understanding moved through me. It was impossible and too much yet I stayed. That's the gift of the medicines, the gift of capacitation. I've been longing to marry the love that is unbounded, the love that is all around us and in us with this inexplicable humanness we bear. I've longed to understand how it can be both. Yesterday I sat at both places. I wept and felt and I stayed in willingness and desire, I stayed in that exact exquisite place of union of un-manifest and manifest, love and humanity. Mark Nepo has written, "I am so sad and everything is beautiful." It was that times a thousand, times a million. I saw how life is all of that we are open to. If we choose awareness, awakeness, if we choose love and life. Some are just able to live at that juncture, somehow are born with that grace, or they learned it somehow. I had no good guide. I've come to it through sheer necessity. I have had teachers and angels, yes, absolutely, and means, of course. And probably cosmic convergence. I'm not saying I'm proud of myself. I'm saying I'm grateful. For all that has conspired to bring me to this place. To this medicine. To this healing.

Male / 28 / USA / Doctorate student

My eating disorder started in my teens. The pressure for guys to look good sent me on that path. Plus, we had a lot of family issues growing up in my house. What I learned later is it is a feeling that I have control. I can control what goes and stays in my body. Since I couldn't really control anything else in my life really.

There was an ad for volunteers with eating disorders to join a study. I was sick of having this controlling my life, so I applied. The medicine they used was ketamine in combination with therapy. Spoiler alert; I can say it was life changing for me. There were many sessions of therapy and ketamine by IV with therapy. The ketamine created an awareness in myself I have never felt. I had empathy and love toward myself and my body. It was something I couldn't have EVER imagined. It was a snowball downhill effect. The better feelings I felt, the less anxious I was. The less anxious I was, the less depressed I was. Each session was different. I don't know if they changed the dose but the last session I had, I literally felt like I was going to die and then I did. But I didn't and for some reason, that gave me the gift of seeing how precious my life was. It helped me to realize how much I want to really live my life in happiness and joy. It's only been about a year but if I start going downhill again, you can bet that I will be running to the closest clinic.

Female / 61 / California / Model

Rehab failed me twice. The craving just wouldn't go away. The bottle was always calling me to it. My marriage was about to end if I couldn't get a grip. A family member who had recently secretly been doing psychedelics for her depression came out to me. She told me to keep it between us because no one knew. But she told me this because she thought it could help me. I talked to my psychiatrist about it and he recommended Ketamine since it's the only legal psychedelic right now with that kind of healing potential. It's pretty expensive and you need at least 6 sessions (they recommend). But it is not an all-day thing. The process takes about an hour total. Then I go see my psychiatrist for another hour.

After the first 4 sessions the craving mostly left me. I wasn't thinking about it constantly. Thanks be to God!! I am not just depending on this to 'cure' me. I still see my psychiatrist and attend my AA meetings. I have been reading that there are places that are doing therapy when you are under Ketamine. I will be researching that but my plan is to continue the Ketamine sessions however I can make it happen and see how my future unfolds.

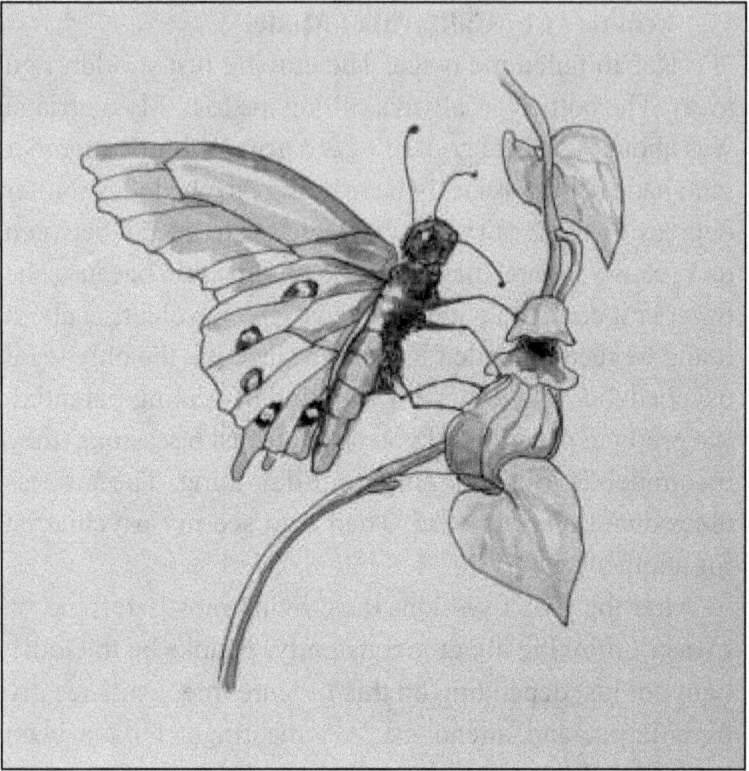

STORIES OF HEALING WITH MICRODOSING

Research has shown that even small doses of psychedelics can help build new neural connections, which has led to the popularity of microdosing. A microdose is defined as any amount below the psychoactive threshold, typically ranging from 1/5 to 1/20 of a standard psychedelic dose used for a full session. The specific amount depends on various factors, such as the substance itself, a person's weight, and their sensitivity level. The goal of microdosing is to remain sub-perceptual, meaning the dose isn't strong enough to cause hallucinations. Microdosing is not about "tripping"; instead, it allows a person to go about their regular day fully present and coherent.

Microdosing is often used to promote heightened focus and productivity, boost creativity, and support mental health conditions such as depression and anxiety. Some people also microdose for general well-being, experiencing gradual health improvements over time. The benefits of microdosing typically develop over several weeks or months. People appreciate microdosing for its slow and gentle effects, as opposed to a full psychedelic dose, which may work more quickly but can be intimidating for some. Microdosing can also serve as a gentle introduction to a substance or help extend the healing effects after a larger psychedelic experience.

Dr. Conor Murray, Ph.D., from UCLA's Semel Institute, conducted a placebo-controlled study in which low doses of LSD were administered to healthy adults to observe the effects on reward-related brain activity—a response often diminished in depression. The surprising result was that, even when participants couldn't tell they had taken the drug, the small dose still enhanced brain activity. The takeaway? There may be a "sweet spot" where microdosing sharpens brain function without altering perception. Dr. Murray predicts that microdosing, rather than large doses, may offer the greatest benefits for brain health and wellness.

Different philosophies exist regarding microdosing schedules. The most common is the protocol developed by Dr. James Fadiman, a prominent psychologist and researcher trained at Stanford. Dr. Fadiman conducted studies until 1966 when research was halted, but later sought to standardize microdosing for more consistent research outcomes. Over the years, he has collected reports from people in more than 80 countries who have microdosed. Fadiman discovered that combining microdosing with talk therapy greatly enhances its effectiveness, while also revealing microdosing's benefits for pain relief.

Both Dr. Fadiman and Paul Stamets have developed microdosing protocols, recommending a schedule of microdosing for about a month, with breaks in between rather than daily use. From university lectures to features in outlets like *The New York Times*, microdosing has become a widely discussed and increasingly popular topic.

LSD, SAN PEDRO, AND PSILOCYBIN MICRODOSING STORIES

Male / 29 / Canada / Athlete

After a pretty bad brain injury playing hockey the team doctor was trying all of the traditional treatments for recovery. Canada now is doing some alternative medicines and my parents thought it might be worth a try. My mom grew up in the 60's in San Francisco CA so she knew all about psychedelics. Studies are showing that LSD and other types of these psychedelics are growing synopsis and making new pathways in the brain. The whole brain plasticity science at its best. My mom found a place that would take me on as a patient. There was a lot involved. I just didn't go in and take something. There were talk appointments, tests to track progress, writing in a booklet every day. Plus, I continued with the team doctor and all of those treatments.

The microdose is a 10th of a normal dose and I take it every 4th day. I never noticed any tripping or anything like that. It has been 2 years now and my brain is better than ever. Everyone agrees that I should stop now and see what happens. The consensus is that the brain won't go back after the work is done. So, please pray for me and my brain.

Female / 39 / Alberta / Surgeon

For years, I quietly listened to women in integration groups discussing their psychedelic experiences. I read extensively on the subject and tried every self-help modality imaginable to heal my performance anxiety. The idea of taking a large dose was terrifying and caused me severe anxiety just thinking about it. During this time, the topic of microdosing frequently came up. Although it was said to be a slow process, people reported it as a steady path to healing.

I was torn between taking the slow approach or facing my fears and undertaking a significant journey. Ultimately, I decided to microdose. It was the right decision for me, as the process involved far less stress and anxiety about what might happen. I stopped feeling self-pressure to take large doses like most others.

After a slow and steady 13 months of following the James Fadiman protocol, I am pleased to report that my anxiety has substantially diminished. The progress was gradual, with breaks in between known as integration time. Initially, the changes were barely noticeable, but reading my journals from six months to three years ago, it's amazing how much better I am now. Sometimes I wonder how I managed my job with the constant anxiety I used to feel. Today, I am confident in my abilities to help others as a physician.

Male / 66 / California / Non-disclosed

I REALLY don't want to be identified BUT the experience I had microdosing LSD has literally changed my personality. And hopefully by me telling my story, it can change someone else for the better if they have the guts to try it. I shouldn't say it that way because the hardest part was making the decision to try it. In my teenage years, we were told it would fry your brain so it put a fear in me to take any kind of drug. But taking the microdose ended up being so easy and painless. Except for a calming, peaceful effect I wouldn't have known I was doing anything. It helped my awareness BEFORE I spouted off or got angry. So, I would know it was coming, not like the anger was just a volcano spewing unexpectedly. I also felt more productive in a good way. Which made me feel better about myself. I think that lowered my reasons for being so angry.

Two microdosing sessions a month apart went by and between time, it seems to be sticking. My coach has me following Fadiman's book and guidelines. Wait a month and start again. With just this month I can feel I am a better person. But that is just step ten and I want to be at step 100 someday. And the great thing is that I truly feel that I can be at 100 someday.

Male / 40 / Midland, TX / Veteran

Two tours didn't do me any favors. After that, I decided to become a civilian again. A civilian who had PTSD. Life at home was hard. Nothing I did seemed important. Everything I did seemed hard. By chance I started renting a house from a woman who was a psychedelic integration coach. To cut to the chase, she recommended microdosing mushrooms. People think that more is better (all the big sessions with psychedelics). She convinced me otherwise. I am on my 4th round. One month on every third day then two months off. Life goes on as usual. It is not noticeable as far as a 'high'. What is noticeable is that my PTSD has consistently been fading away. Life to me is precious now. Everything I do seems important in one way or another. And life seems so much easier. This has been a Godsend for me and most likely a life saver because I wouldn't want to have lived much longer the way I was living. Crazy that this isn't legal and that really pisses me off. The chance I am taking using this in Texas is a possible prison sentence. But better than a death sentence of living with PTSD.

Female / 39 / Miami, FL / Sales Associate

After a serious trauma my body has been in pain for years. Doctors don't know if it was all in my head or actually physical. At any rate, I lived in tremendous pain that was almost unbearable. That along with the trauma was making me literally go wacky. Thank goodness someone led me down the psychedelic mushroom microdosing path. It wasn't magic, the work still needs to be done in combination. But I will tell you from my experience that they are a lifesaver if used with respect and intentionally. It has been equal to decades of therapy, testing, research, prescriptions and all the other things I have tried combined. I am not suggesting people are miraculously healed forever. Life is an ongoing project where we work on ourselves. But with the microdosing and not all the prescriptions, I am without side effects that the medications were giving me. And I don't have any perceptible feelings other than seeing my pain lessen as time goes on. Every day I feel more and more like my old self and can see my old life coming back into reach.

Male / 79 / Florida / Pet Store Owner

For years I had struggled with emotional pain. In my day, men just pulled themselves up by their bootstraps and didn't complain or talk about it. Then on top of it as I started aging, my body was in daily pain even though my business kept me pretty active. One day during a checkup I decided to mention the emotional pain I had been struggling with for years. My doctor suggested ketamine sessions to help with the emotional pain I had and temporarily help with the physical pain. It was a very long drive for me to the clinic he recommended but after seeing that it was helping after several sessions, it was suggested I take it at home as a lozenge. Slow and steady was how they put it. Any progress for me would be welcome at that point. The therapist put me on a regiment and told me that more was not better. If the low dose was working don't bump it up. As the weeks went by, I noticed my brain was calmer, more open to just let shit go and I was in less pain. The intention was to help my mind, the pain recession was a very welcome side effect. It isn't something that should be done constantly or for long periods of time so I take a break per the doctor's recommendations. Hopefully, I can stop altogether in the near future.

It is just a nice helping hand for now.

Female / 63 / USA / Retired

I have been microdosing for about a year and 1/2 now. First mushrooms, then LSD and then San Pedro. I heard that all 3 were amazing consistent healers. I tried mushrooms for 30 days then took about 6 weeks off to compare microdosing with LSD. Then LSD for about 20 days but it seemed to make me forget words even at ½ of a microdose. So maybe LSD is not the one for me. San Pedro brought me awareness. I have finished a 30-day session twice several months apart. The slow and steady process is good for me. No slap in the face like with a large dose experience which is fine by me. Journalling is a must so I can watch my progress and record my ah-ha moments of realization. The weird thing is on microdose day, it seems someone challenges me in the area that I am working on. It gives me awareness and a bit of space to respond and not react which is very helpful.

Female / 59 / Central Valley, CA / Truck Driver

There were years of suffering from pain from a long past injury. I tried physical therapy, pain killers (over the counter and prescription), yoga and surgery. But nothing helped. Driving an 18-wheeler on long haul trips doesn't help. One evening I was in conversation with another driver and he mentioned that he was microdosing LSD. He said he could still drive and it was not detectable, he felt perfectly normal. His claim was that it took away the pain. Generously he gave me enough for two weeks and explained the protocol. I got his number in case it worked and he could let me know how to get more. It was about

2 times more than a traditional microdose according to authorities but still 1/8th of a regular dose. The crazy thing is that it worked! After reading more about LSD and how it works in/on the brain. I still didn't have the 'why' understanding but I am not a scientist so a lot of it sounded weird, but I don't care because it is the only thing to ever work for me!

Female / 66 / Redlands, CA / Music Teacher

After retiring, I fell into a depression—or at least I think that's what it was. I felt stuck, unable to commit or make decisions about anything. My job had been my life, and suddenly, I had no purpose. One day at the library, I stumbled upon a book featuring works by people like Freud and Gower. It was fascinating because it discussed how the brain functions while also offering philosophical quotes that resonated with me.

Then, by chance, I came across a podcast interview with a famous neurologist who was researching psychedelics. He reiterated a lot of the information I had just read about the brain. As I listened, I realized the conversation was essentially describing what was happening in my own mind.

So, I reached out to a few old friends—former hippies—and asked if they knew anything about psychedelics or had access to them. Of course, they did. They connected me with a wonderful woman who was doing underground work with LSD. She recommended that I have several talk sessions with her to identify my needs and the issues I was struggling with. After two sessions, we both felt comfortable moving forward with microdosing LSD. The plan was to microdose for one month, followed by another session to assess progress. She provided me with thorough instructions, and off I went.

The first day I took it, I felt nothing, just as she had said would be the goal—but it was still working on my brain. By the third dose, my days started to feel easier, brighter, and I found myself more able to make decisions. As the month went on, I felt increasingly better, even though I still didn't feel any physical effects. After our session at the end of that first month, we decided to continue for two more months. The transformation was remarkable! By the end of the third month, my brain and emotions were in a much better place.

During our next session, we revisited the reasons why I had sought help in the first place, and most of those issues had significantly improved. As she had mentioned from the start, microdosing was not meant to be a permanent, ongoing treatment. I was to take a three-month break and then check in with her. During the break, I continued journaling, exercising, and engaging in other activities that were good for me.

Now, eight months after starting microdosing, I feel like my old self again. Retirement is great, and I no longer feel lost. It's as if I've found the map that guides me in this new chapter of my life. I'm not sure if I'll microdose again, but I would certainly consider it if I needed to. It's amazing how such a tiny amount of something like LSD can change a person's brain—and attitude.

Female / 29 / Omaha, Nebraska / Emergency Room Doctor

I had heard about psychedelic healing for a long time. I wasn't sure if it was the right avenue for me but they didn't make me nervous because I have never seen a psychedelic overdose in the ER. What I did need to know was how they actually worked in the brain since I LOVE my brain and didn't want to do anything to harm it. On Spotify, I found several podcasts. One was with Dr. Huberman interviewing Robin Carhart-Harris. It was enough to make the decision to do it.

It was time to get off SSRIs because I didn't like how they made me feel. When I started bringing up the conversation with colleagues, I was immediately hooked up with an underground psychedelic therapist. She recommended I wean off the SSRIs during a vacation. It just so happened I needed to take a family leave to help with a grandparent so I had six weeks off. The first three I weaned off which was scary in of itself. Following my intuition, our zoom therapy sessions and her suggestion, we decided to try microdosing mushrooms. It would be something I could do while still helping with my grandma. And there wouldn't be a 'recovery' period. Starting with a very low microdose, we slowly raised it until I felt the substance. Then we backed it down again to the previous dosage.

Within a little over a week, I felt like I was back on the SSRIs as far as being stable but I still had feelings. Not the numbness I was feeling. It was a beautiful experience because I was able to process what was happening in my life and the illness and death of my grandma. If I wouldn't have had the help of the microdosing, I may have gone into a depression. It has been six months and I am still doing a protocol that Paul Stamets recommends. It is helping me with being able to access old wounds and feelings. I am able to release them and heal a lot of my issues. Too bad this isn't legal because it could be helping so many people and maybe stopping some of the attempted suicides I see coming into the ER.

Female / 36 / Melbourne / Nurse

I started a San Pedro microdosing regimen for several reasons. I also joined a local community to learn more and connect with others using psychedelics. It has been a year now doing it. A lot of things have changed for me very silently and slowly but with great progress. But the most interesting thing I would like to mention in this healing story is that my issue with trichotillomania (compulsive hair pulling) has lessened to almost zero (strange it took me some time to notice). Maybe it was because it was so slow and I was doing it less and less. Then one day I was aware that it had stopped. This was a 24+ year habit.

What a gift that I didn't consciously ask for!!

Female / 68 / Tucson / Retired Airline Employee

Microdosing with psilocybin brought me deep feelings of calm, peace, gratitude, creativity and generosity. I also noted a lot of productivity, not always about getting a lot of things done, but also making decisions that I had been putting off. I often felt like I was "in the flow". Insights were downloading, nothing so very profound necessarily, but rather a sense of settling in, integrating, really knowing what I know. -If that makes sense. I also felt an acute sense of wonder and awe -even in the mundane.

Microdosing with San Pedro, very early on I noted that I felt like I could warp time. It felt like everything that needed to get done, got done, but without striving or stressing. I guess that is what being in the flow means. I was also aware of synchronicities happening all around me, all of the time it seemed. New opportunities presented themselves. I had very detailed lucid dreams, and I felt amazing and exhilarated. I was also aware of the beauty of creation and of prayers being answered.

Even after I finished both protocols, I was still aware of insights settling in. Now I am getting eager for another round since it has been almost a year!

Male / 68 / Washington / Retired Real Estate

Since I was nervous for my health and taking a big dose, it was suggested I try microdosing San Pedro. This made me more comfortable. Especially since it wasn't going to even be a 'high'. I actually didn't even notice that I had taken anything except that I felt calmer and everything seemed so much easier. I guess you would call it a flow state. Things just came together without me 'having' to control everything. And I didn't have any anxiety because I didn't have to have control. So far, I did 3 different months over the course of a year. With several months in between the month that I was microdosing. I will continue on this path as it seems to work for me in my healing path. Less anxiety, life is easier and a little less OCD.

Female / 44 / Sydney, Australia / Manager

Since I was about 14, I have been struggling with hormones and moods. Some years were much worse than others. After 3 children, it seemed it was getting worse from the stress of raising 3 active kids and working full time.

By chance I came upon a women's psychedelic group when on vacation in Adelaide. They generously let me sit in and that was the start of my journey. Listening to other women telling their stories of how microdosing helped with regulating their hormones better than prescriptions changed my future. I was able to get connected with someone who could help me with the process pretty easily even though she was doing it underground. After 3 rounds, I am feeling enormous relief from my symptoms. My doctor wasn't so sure about it when I reported it to her. BUT, I know myself and what is working for me so I will continue until it no longer works or I no longer need it. I thank these medicines from the bottom of my heart as well as my husband and kids are very appreciative!!!

Female / 47 / Nevada / Travel Nurse

Encouraged by my life coach who knew my history with men and bad relationships, I started microdosing. We tried several different psychedelics to see which one was right for me. First LSD for one month. A month off, then Ketamine. After another month off, I tried microdosing mushrooms. That turned out to be a good fit for me. It has been several years with large stretches of time in between. When I feel it's time, I start again for a month or two. Looking back over old journals, I can see how much it has changed my life. Incredible! Slow but very steady. Mostly so slow that it was hard to notice until I looked back. Reading old journals actually was very depressing that I was living in that headspace. Which is why my life coach probably thought it would help. I couldn't be more grateful for being steered that direction. I know I felt better, just didn't realize how much better! I found love and respect for my deserving self and realized I only deserved loving caring treatment from others.

Female / 67 / Oregon / Retired Dental Office Manager

While microdosing San Pedro I noticed several things. But first I would like to say that it took a bit of time to get the dosing right. If the dose was a little higher, it would make me tired. If the dose was too low, I didn't notice any changes in my day. When the amount was clearly right, it was wonderful. I had so much more focus. The fuzzy brain and the ADHD I diagnosed myself with seemed to retreat. It helped me to be more aware of 'the now' and not constantly hopping from one thing to the next and back.

Yes! I would recommend it. And be patient until you find your proper dosing.

Female / 24 / Texas / Medical School Student

I put so much pressure on myself to do perfect in everything. It started to make me feel like I was cracking up. Anxiety, procrastination and sleeplessness started creeping into my days. Which wasn't me at all. My roommate told me that she met a psychedelic integration coach and she was starting to microdose mushrooms. She was also feeling very anxious trying to 'keep up'. I met with this coach and had a talk session with her and we came up with a plan for me. This was over a year ago and I have been working with her since. We have made several adjustments and taken time off between the months I microdosed. Even though they were off months, I still felt the mushrooms were in me, guiding me. It truly is a living wise plant. I am so grateful that this came into my life. It's scary to me to see the road I was going down. I probably would have needed heavy medication if it continued.

The thing is, that wouldn't have healed me, this route is healing me and that makes me so grateful.

Female / 66 / La Jolla / Business Owner

This was so out of my realm! A friend who has experience in these things came out to me about doing it. It took a while but I started asking questions which she generously shared. Finally, she said she would help me get some mushrooms and guide me on the way microdosing should be done. She encouraged me to journal, join a group of women who were also doing this for healing and try to have some quiet time every day.

After 30 days of doing it the way she recommended, I could already see some changes. It was very surprising to me and so very easy. My dull moods started shifting, I could feel more times of happiness and awe. It's strange because even a month after I have completed that round, I still feel like I am continuing the healing process. When it feels right and the healing feeling slows down, I will welcome trying another round. It was so different than I expected. For some reason (probably all the propaganda I grew up with about psychedelics) I was apprehensive about being "high" but except for feeling better, I felt nothing else. It wasn't even like drinking a glass of wine.

Female / 45 / Dana Point, CA / Specialist for kids with autism

Well first I will say if my employer found out, it would be the end of my career working with kids so it was a HUGE step for me. I suffered from multiple female issues probably due to the stress I put on myself. I never had children but not because of that. So many days spent in pain. One evening, I saw a news report about people microdosing psychedelics and started thinking, "well nothing else has worked...". So, I discreetly started asking around and googling information. Praying the whole time that I wouldn't be 'tracked' by doing that. Even though I did the searches incognito. As it turns out a friend opened up that she was also looking into it. Luckily for both of us, she found an avenue.

After two 30-day microdosing regimes, I noticed my pain was much less. Slowly better and my biggest surprise was that I could still drive, function and work without ANY indication I had taken something. I don't know scientifically how it works but it has. I have found a very small local community of women to compare notes and support each other. When I feel that the pain has stopped going away, I will absolutely do another round. But since it still is slowly working, I don't feel the need.

Male / 81 / Phoenix, AZ / Retired Military

My grandfather came to live with me after his dementia got too bad to be alone. He also developed sundown syndrome, meaning he would be up pacing all night, which left both of us sleep-deprived—I was constantly worried he might leave the house. Then, out of nowhere, he slept through the night for three nights in a row. It felt strange when he didn't wake me up because I had become so used to it.

That's when I discovered he had gotten into my microdosing stash. When I asked him about it, he thought they were his medications and had unknowingly been taking them for those three nights. Curious to see if there was a connection, I decided to give him another dose on the fourth day. Miraculously, he slept through the night again. This continued for a month, and I couldn't believe the difference.

I started to wonder if we needed to take a break, since you're not typically supposed to microdose every day. After skipping it for two nights, he was back to waking up at night. At that point, I figured, why not? He's 81, not in great shape, and if this drug-free method helps him sleep, then it's worth it. Mind you, regular sleeping pills had never worked when I tried those.

Now, he microdoses every day, and it continues to work. If it ever stops, I'll consider adjusting the amount. I haven't come across any studies on this, but it doesn't matter much—he's become my own case study, and the results have been nothing short of a miracle. With him getting more sleep, his cognition is much better now also.

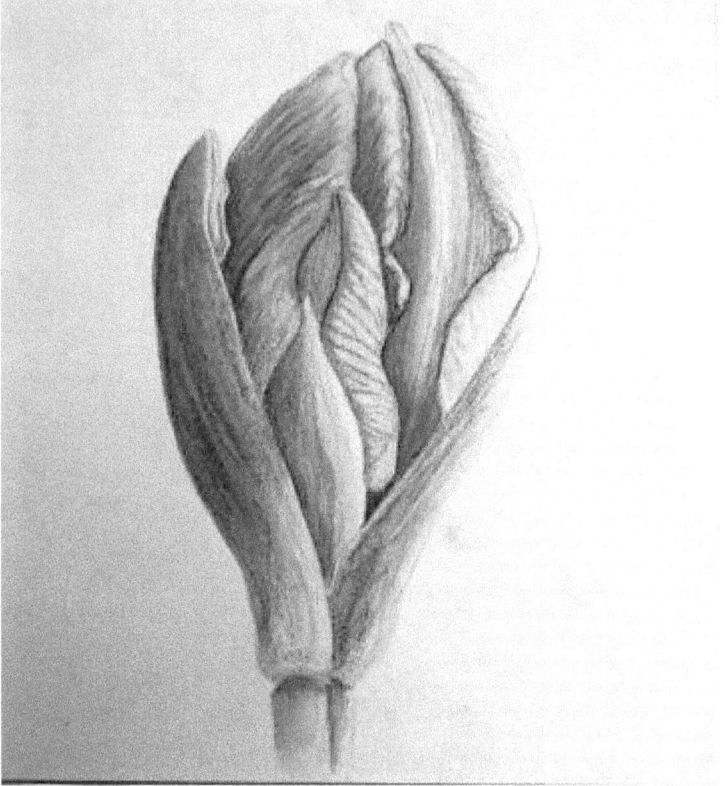

CONCLUSION

"What a wonderful thought it is that some of the best days of our lives haven't even happened yet."

-Anne Frank

Now that you've read these stories of healing with psychedelics, let's take a moment to reflect on common themes. This book features numerous accounts of six different substances, each one addressing unique challenges experienced by your average, every day citizen. Individuals who could be your neighbor, doctor, or child's school teacher.

Take the workforce trainer, for example, who used psilocybin to heal from C-PTSD and ADHD. Or the barista who found relief from chronic migraines through use of psilocybin. A rancher who was finally able to quit smoking and take better care of his body after his experience with mushrooms.

In the accounts of mescaline, we saw a business owner experience a profound heart-opening transformation, while a neurologist discovered a newfound love for herself, others, and the planet. Ayahuasca stories revealed many powerful insights as well, such as the stay at-home father who realized he had been living in a constant state of fight, flight, or freeze without even being aware of why. Or the retired man who worried that Ayahuasca might compromise his sobriety, but instead found it freed him from his desire to drink and helped alleviate his depression.

Those who tried LSD reported improvements in temper, frustration, and feelings of disconnection. One preschool teacher, in particular, expressed how she regained control over her mind and thoughts, crediting LSD for her sanity. A story of MDMA use emphasized how it strengthened two couples' marriage, while Ketamine helped a tattoo artist overcome postpartum depression. A doctoral student also attributed Ketamine with helping him manage his eating disorder. The benefits of microdosing were also made clear as it provided healing for a number of participants: an athlete recovering from a brain injury, a nurse who was able to quit her compulsive hairpulling, and a surgeon who experienced a significant reduction in anxiety.

These stories ultimately reveal how psychedelics helped people heal from a number of debilitating issues when other forms of treatment failed them. With countless reports of healing worldwide, it's time we start listening to these stories with open hearts and encourage others to do the same. There is still so much stigma and shame surrounding psychedelic use, despite the growing body of evidence—both anecdotal and scientific—that demonstrates their healing potential.

If someone you care about is exploring a different path to healing, you can show support by asking questions, seeking to understand, and reading more about this topic. Countless medical professionals and studies have shed light on how these substances impact the brain and why they work. I invite you to keep an open heart and mind and celebrate these individuals who are finding healing, even if their chosen path feels unfamiliar to you.

If you found this book insightful or meaningful, I would be grateful if you could leave a review on Amazon or wherever you purchased it. Your feedback helps others who may benefit from these stories find the book more easily and contributes to the ongoing conversation around psychedelic healing.

Thank you for your support!

Every healing journey is unique. Even with the same dose of the same medicine, experiences and outcomes vary greatly due to individual circumstances. Attempting to replicate someone else's experience is not advised. The courageous individuals mentioned in this book approached their journeys with intention, education, and collaboration. They combined their experiences with practices like journaling, meditation, yoga, and integration groups. Healing is a communal and continuous process, requiring effort and support.

While psychedelic therapy can bring profound insights, it is not a cure-all. These substances may illuminate hidden issues by reducing interference from the ego or critical thinking. However, lasting transformation requires sustained effort, ongoing integration, and professional support. The brain naturally resists change to preserve familiar patterns, prioritizing survival over growth. True healing comes from addressing these patterns and fostering new, healthier ways of being.

Psychedelic experiences carry potential risks, particularly for individuals with certain mental health conditions. If you are considering exploring these substances, consult with medical and psychological professionals to
determine whether it is safe and appropriate for you

DISCLAIMER

This book does not promote or endorse the use of psychedelic substances. Its goal is to educate readers on how these substances can serve as powerful tools for healing when used safely, legally, and intentionally. The potential for individual healing is immense when proper protocols are followed, including setting intentions, creating a safe environment, and working with a trusted guide or licensed therapist.

This book does not constitute professional, legal, or medical advice. The author and contributors are not encouraging readers to engage in dangerous or illegal activities. Readers are advised to research and comply with the laws in their respective jurisdictions regarding psychedelic substances. The author assumes no responsibility for any consequences resulting from the use of information contained herein.

If you or someone you know is in crisis or experiencing a mental health emergency, please seek immediate help. In the U.S., you can call or text 988 to connect with the National Suicide Prevention Lifeline. For international resources, consult local agencies or organizations in your area.

The purpose of this book is solely to initiate a mainstream conversation about these substances and their therapeutic potential

REFERENCES

Barbaro, Michael, et al. "The Veterans Fighting to Legalize Psychedelics." *The New York Times*, 22 Feb. 2023. www.nytimes.com/2023/02/22/podcasts/the-daily/veterans-psychedelics-legalization.html

Dyck, Erika. *Psychedelic Psychiatry: LSD from Clinic to Campus.* Johns Hopkins University Press, 2008.

Hallifax, James. "A Brief History of MDMA: From the CIA to Raves to Psychedelic Therapy." Psychedelic Spotlight, 2 June 2024. psychedelicspotlight.com/history-of-mdma-cia-ravespsychedelic-therapy

Hasty, Marie. "Who Can Benefit from Ketamine Therapy? Psychedelic Support." *Psychedelic Support* , 19 Aug. 2024, psychedelic.support/resources/who-can-benefit-from-ketamine-therapy

Li, Linda, and Phillip E. Vlisides. "Ketamine: 50 Years of Modulating the Mind." *Frontiers in Human Neuroscience* vol. 10 612. 29 Nov. 2016, doi:10.3389/fnhum.2016.00612

Migala Jessica. "What Is Ketamine Therapy? Risks, Benefits, Effectiveness, and More." EverydayHealth.Com, 18 Aug. 2023, www.everydayhealth.com/integrative-health/ketamine-therapy/guide

Saint Thomas, Sophie. "Can Psychedelics Treat Alcohol Use Disorder?" *Psychable*, 20 Oct. 2022. psychable.com/addiction/can-psychedelics-treat-alcoholuse-disorder.

Visser, E. and S.A. Schug. "The Role of Ketamine in Pain Management." *Biomedicine & Pharmacotherapy = Biomedecine & Pharmacotherapie* vol. 60,7 (2006): 341-8. doi:10.1016/j.biopha.2006.06.021

ADDITIONAL RESOURCES

Paul Stamets, Mycologist, is the foremost expert on all kinds of fungi. He has Ted Talks, YouTube videos, books and a website: https://paulstamets.com

Studies at Imperial College in London. Therapeutic use of psychedelics in 1980's to 1990's by a Swiss psychiatrist, Peter Gasser. Using LSD as a tool. He saw notable increased well-being.

Professor Robin Carhart-Harris et al., *"The Paradoxical Psychological Effects of Lysergic Acid Diethylamide (LSD).* There are also an amazing number of YouTube and TED talk videos with Professor Carhart-Harris speaking on psychedelics and healing.

Frontiers in Pharmacology Frontiersin.org

Center for Psychedelic & Consciousness Research. hopkinspsychedelic.org

PMC PubMed Central

The American Psychological Association has reports from top researchers. From Johns Hopkins to Stanford. www.apa.org/education-career/ce/science-psychedelics

Interesting article/study regarding microdosing on PMC PubMed Central; Polito V, Stevenson RJ. A systematic study of microdosing psychedelics. PLoS One. 2019 Feb 6;14(2):e0211023. doi: 10.1371/journal.pone.0211023.

PMID: 30726251; PMCID: PMC6364961.

Healthline.com has an article regarding Ayahuasca for changing the brain. Written by Jillian Kubala, MS, RD — Updated on August 21, 2024

BMC Neuroscience has an extensive paper written on June 30, 2023 called Psychedelics and neural plasticity. https://bmcneurosci.biomedcentral.com/articles/10.1186/s12868-023-00809-0

Clinicaltrials.gov

Duke Researchers Probe the Magic of Psychedelics as Medicine. October 25, 2023 By Dan Vahaba, PhD

Massachusetts General Center for the Neuroscience of Psychedelics. www.massgeneral.org

Google research on psychedelics and you will find hundreds if not thousands of articles by top universities and researchers.

Dr. Gul Dolen is doing research on psychedelics and the brain. dolenlab.org/research

ORGANIZATIONS THAT SUPPORT EDUCATION, COMMUNITY, AND MORE

Multidisciplinary Association for Psychedelic Studies (MAPS) is a leader in psychedelic research. A nonprofit research and educational organization that develops medical, legal and cultural contexts for people to benefit from the careful uses of psychedelics. MAPS currently sponsors some of the most advanced clinical trials and studies worldwide. https://maps.org

Daniel Shankin is the founder and director of Tam Integration He is committed to offering accessible and inclusive support and education for people who are wanting to transform, heal, and grow. Tam's integration circles are hosted on Zoom, making them accessible to everyone. Tamintegration.com

Moms on Mushrooms, created by Tracey Tee, a Colorado mom. This group offers courses, education and community. They are deeply concerned for health and safety. Momsonmushrooms.com

Dedicated to the practice of compassionate and ethical Ketamine assisted psychotherapy, Polaris Insight Center is located in San Francisco. https://www.polarisinsight.com

American Society of Ketamine Physicians, Psychotherapists, and Practitioners (ASKP). This nonprofit group focuses on the safe clinical use of ketamine for mental health disorders and pain conditions. The most useful resource for the public is their directory to help you locate a ketamine physician in your area.

UC Berkeley Center for the Science of Psychedelics. A consumer-friendly website covers the basics of psychedelic therapy, including what psychedelics are, choosing a psychedelic therapist, the risks and how to stay safe, as well as how the legal landscape surrounding these drugs is changing.
https://psychedelics.berkeley.edu

WOOP offers resources to support women on their psychedelic journey. Education, harm reduction, and hosting online and in person events. Their mission is to empower and connect women worldwide on their personal journeys of self-discovery and healing.
https://www.womenonpsychedelics.com

Jesse Gould, a former Army Ranger, was plagued by severe PTSD after he returned home from combat. He found healing using psychedelics and eventually started Heroic Hearts Project to help veterans heal from PTSD. https://heroicheartsproject.org/

A new nonprofit called the Indigenous Peyote Conservation Initiative. www.ipci.life

Almost every country and state have a Psychedelic Society that can provide a community platform focused on education, advocacy and connection.

DOCUMENTARIES AND NEWS REPORTS

Can Psychedelics Cure? Premiered 10/19/22. Top: Body + Brain
https://www.youtube.com/watch?v=4p798ozffHQ

PBS: *How Psychedelics Change The Brain*
www.pbs.org/wgbh/nova/article/spychedelic-brain-effects-claustrum

BBC, *Australia legalizes psychedelics for mental health.*
www.bbc.com/news/world-australia-66072427

How a first responder says MDMA helped him get past PTSD with Eric Sienknecht, PsyD September 2019,
https://www.youtube.com/watch?v=4p798ozffHQ

9
A Conversation about Ketamine assisted Psychotherapy with Veronika Gold, LMFT and Gregory Wells, PhD. January, 2019. https://www.veronikagold.com/media

A movie about taking psychedelics at Dosed.com

ARTICLES

CBS News: Using Psychedelics to Treat Veterans' PTSD. March 27, 2024

https://www.stripes.com/incoming/2024-02-16/veteranspsychedelic-drugs-ptsd-13025296.html

https://www.yahoo.com/news/veterans-turn-psychedelics-mexico-ptsd-131000526.html

https://www.nytimes.com/2024/12/16/us/psychedelicibogaine-veteran-brain-injury-ptsd.html

CBS News: Psilocybin Sessions: Psychedelics Could Help People with Addictions and Anxiety with Anderson Cooper 10/13/2019
https://www.cbsnews.com/news/psychedelic-drugs-lsd-Forbes: MDMA-Assisted Therapy for PTSD: Science Behind the Hype. January 29, 2024
https://www.forbes.com/sites/sarahsin-clair/2024/03/27/mdma-assisted-therapy-for-ptsd-thehistory-and-science-behind-the-hype/

UC Berkeley for the Science of Psychedelics
https://psychedelics.berkeley.edu/resources/psychiatricre
search-with-hallucinogens-what-have-we-learned

From the NY Times; This is Literally Your Brain on
Drugs
https://www.nytimes.com/2024/07/17/health/psilocybin-
psychedelic-mushroomsbrain.html?smid=em=share

Londoño E. "After Six-Decade Hiatus, Experimental
Psychedelic Therapy Returns to the V.A.". New York
Times. 06/24/2022.

How do psychedelics work? A report on NOVA
https://www.pbs.org/wgbh/nova/article/psychedelicbrain-effects-claustrum

Ketamine Assisted Psychotherapy (KAP): Patient Demographics, Clinical Data and Outcomes in Three Large Practices Administering Ketamine with Psychotherapy. Full article: Ketamine Assisted Psychotherapy (KAP): Patient Demographics, Clinical Data and Outcomes in Three Large Practices Administering Ketamine with Psychotherapy. www.tandfonline.com

Ketamine for the treatment of major depression
https://www.thelancet.com/journals/eclinm/article/PIIS2589-5370(23)00304-8/fulltext

Ketamine as an antidepressant.
https://pmc.ncbi.nlm.nih.gov/articles/PMC7225830

Can Psychedelics Treat Alcohol Use Disorder? Sophie Saint Thomas 4/23/2021 Medical Editor: Dr. Benjamin Malcolm, PharmD, MPH, BCPP Phycable.

BOOKS

How To Change Your Mind by Michael Pollan (2018): Pollan combines personal narrative with scientific research, documenting his own journey of exploration and shedding light on the therapeutic potential of psychedelics. There has also been a Netflix documentary made with the same name.

Microdosing For Health, Healing and Enhanced Performance, by Dr. Jim Fadiman (2025)

LSD And the Mind of The Universe by Christopher Bache

Listening to Ayahuasca and *Swimming in the Sacred,* both by Rachael Harris PHD

A Really Good Day by Ayelet Waldman: Waldman's memoir recounts her experiences with microdosing, exploring the impact of small doses of psychedelics on her mood and well-being.

Realms of The Human Unconscious by Stanislav Grof.

Sacred Knowledge by William A. Richards (2015): Richards, a seasoned researcher, presents an in-depth examination of the spiritual and transformative aspects of psychedelic experiences, drawing upon his extensive work with individuals undergoing psychedelic-assisted therapy.

The Psychedelics Explorer's Guide by James Fadiman (2011): Fadiman provides practical guidance and insights for those interested in safely and responsibly exploring psychedelic substances, drawing on his vast knowledge and experience in the field.

Additionally, numerous books have been authored by medical doctors, researchers and scientists offering comprehensive explorations of the effects of psychedelics on the brain and mind.

SOCIAL MEDIA

Andrew Huberman is an American neuroscientist who has a podcast and YouTube channel where he speaks on the healing psychedelics frequently.

Joe Rogan frequently interviews experts in the field of psychedelics on his podcast. https://www.joerogan.com

Double Blind started as a print magazine and turned into a very successful YouTube Channel and now a podcast. Shelby Hartman is the co-founder and CEO. Madison Margolin is a co-founder and editorial director. Their vision is to educate the public on safe use of psychedelics. Doubleblindmag.com

Paul F. Austin is the founder and CEO of Third Wave. It has a blog, podcasts on Spotify and Apple and a

YouTube channel on psychedelics that connects you to the leaders and pioneers of the psychedelic renaissance. https://thethirdwave.co/

Dr. Tracey Marks, psychiatrist. Her mission is to increase mental health awareness and understanding by education. Watch her on her YouTube

Spirit Pharmacist. Dr. Ben Malcolm PharmD, MPH. Focusing on consultation services and courses on psychedelic healing and pharmacology. He is helping people develop safe and optimum ways to explore psychedelics. Spiritpharacist.com

Radiolab is on a curiosity bender. They ask deep questions and use investigative journalism to get the answers. Radiolab podcast with Molly Webster Radiolab@wnyc.org

For a great video on MDMA explained in an easy-to-understand format. Watch; https://www.spiritpharmacist.com/blog?tag=ptsd

Multidisciplinary Association for Psychedelic Studies (MAPS) Rick Doblin, PhD. Watch his *Origin Story* and his TED Talk.

ADVOCACY GROUPS

Urban Indigenous Collective, founded by Sutton King who is an Indigenous rights activist who's out to transform the culture around psychedelics. She is also calling on science labs to hire Indigenous people as researchers and clinicians. And to encourage pharmaceutical companies to recruit Native Americans to serve on their boards. The history of psychedelics is littered with stories of exploitation and cultural appropriation. And it's prompted important questions as these plant medicines gain mainstream acceptance. https://urbanindigenouscollective.org

People of Color Psychedelic Collective. A non-profit that brings education to people of color and partnering with many other psychedelic societies around the U.S. pocpc.org

Charcruna is an organization that promotes reciprocity in the psychedelic community and supports the protection of sacred plants and cultural traditions. Their mission is to advance psychedelic justice through curating critical conversations and uplisting voices of women, queer people, Indigenous peoples, people of color and the Global South in the field of psychedelic science. They also focus on goals to bridge the gap between the traditions of plant medicines and the emergent field of psychedelic science. Between traditional ceremonial use and clinical and therapeutic settings. As well as focusing on harm reduction. Charcruna.net

The Zendo project's goal is harm reduction. They have training that provides education on how to work with challenging experiences and create a platform for honest and responsible conversations about substance use. Our intention is to create public awareness around the potential risks of drug use and to reduce these risks by providing tools and information. Zendoproject.org

Fireside Project is a group that promotes safety and awareness. They also will assist with psychedelic help if one is having a hard time. Firesideproject.org

Psychedelic Support brings together a network of therapists, counselors, holistic doctors and mainstream medical doctors to offer services (online and in-person) for psychedelic/plant medicine integration, preparation, psychological and physical health and personal growth. https://psychedelic.support

PMC is engaged in federal and state-level efforts to increase access to sponsored research & development efforts. They engage in conversations with federal stakeholders to spur the creation of federal dollars for clinical psychedelic research studies for industry and universities. https://www.psychedelicmedicinecoalition.org

Students for Sensible Drug Policies. In over 300 campuses nationwide. Trying to make changes from campus to the United Nations. Replacing policies rooted in evidence, compassion and human rights. SSDP.org

BIOPHARMACEUTICAL COMPANIES

ATAI Life Sciences is a clinical-stage biopharmaceutical company aiming to transform the treatment of mental health disorders, with offices in New York, San Diego and Berlin. Our vision is to heal mental health disorders so that everyone everywhere can live a more fulfilled life. https://atai.life/contact

Compass Pathways, a biotechnology company dedicated to working to create transformative therapies for those who are not helped by current treatments. Compasspathways.com

Mindmed biopharmaceutical company is conducting worldwide clinical studies. Mindmed.com

ABOUT THE AUTHOR

Alisa is committed to reducing the stigma and judgment surrounding psychedelics, despite cultural and legal barriers. Aiming to encourage open conversations and reduce the secrecy that often surrounds the topic. She believes this is an essential subject deserving of widespread acceptance and understanding and is determined to contribute to its recognition and acceptance.

She has found a new passion in the psychedelic community. A supporter of several psychedelic organizations. She enjoys filling in as a facilitator for people who identify as women integration group to support others on their journeys.

www.ingramcontent.com/pod-product-compliance
Lightning Source LLC
Chambersburg PA
CBHW062057270326
41931CB00013B/3113